Deadly S.N.A.F.U.

**Marine Corps Base Camp
Lejeune**

And

Joint Base Pearl Harbor-

Hickam

Deadly S.N.A.F.U.

MARINE CORPS BASE CAMP LEJEUNE,
NORTH CAROLINA

AND

JOINT BASE PEARL HARBOR-HICKAM,
HAWAII

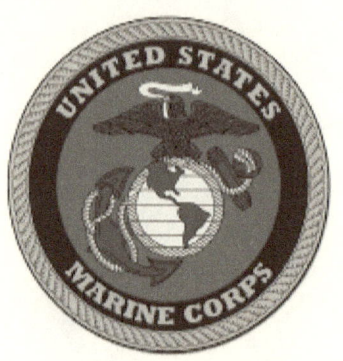

BY

GEORGE SWIMMER

United States Marine Corps Active Reserves,
May 1965 -May 1971 (stationed at Marine Corps Base
Camp Lejeune, North Carolina)

Deadly S.N.A.F.U., Marine Corps Base Camp Lejeune and Joint Base Pearl Harbor-Hickam

Author George Swimmer

ISBN: 9798641618036

Imprint: Independently published

First Edition, June 2020

Second Edition, July 2020

Third Edition, February 2021, Chapter Toxic Vapor Intrusions Didn't End in 1987! Added

Fourth Edition, June 2022, Joint Base Pearl Harbor-Hickam added

In Memoriam

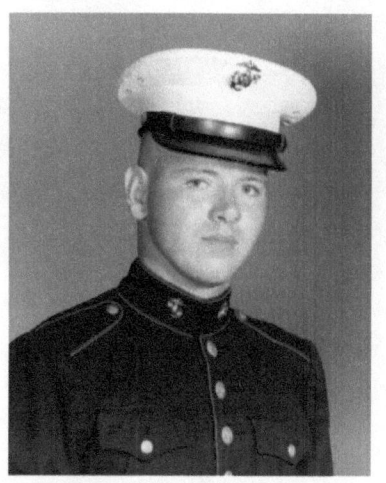

James Charles Rogers

26 APRIL, 1944 – 27 OCTOBER, 2016

Beverly Rogers is a dear friend and the widow of my best friend Jim Rogers. Jim and I had been best friends for almost 60 years; in high school, in the Marines and until he died in 2016. Bev helped me by editing this book and my first book. The following comments are hers.

Bev's comments were made after reading an early edition of the book.

There are sections in this manuscript that address the many health issues faced by children.

Beverly Rogers comments:

I shake my head and wonder how this country allowed a cover up like this to linger so long. Like you, I am angry that this took place. In my mind there is no doubt that Jim's kidney cancer was tied to Camp

Lejeune as well as his Barrett's Esophagus. Yet, these diseases did not appear until much later in his life so for that I am grateful. For many others, this was not the case. Some diseases appeared early in their childhood and ended their lives much too early, breaking the hearts of their parents and family. For others, their family members had to watch while their loved ones suffered through their last years with conditions caused by this poisoned water. How do the officials of the US Marine Corps, Department of the Navy and the Department of Defense live with themselves?

Contents

PROLOGUE I

"OH, WHAT A TANGLED WEB WE WEAVE, WHEN FIRST WE PRACTICE TO DECEIVE!" (SIR WALTER SCOTT, 1808)..1

CAMP LEJEUNE...21

MARINES I SERVED WITH......................26

LETTER AND RESPONSES 34

MORE LIKELY THAN NOT 48

TIMELINE...64

HIDDEN FACTS 77

VICTIMS TESTIFY   82

   Mike Partain   82

   Commander James L. Watters   83

   Peter Devereux   87

THE EXPERT   88

   Dr. Richard Clapp   88

   Michael Hargett   90

THE GOVERNMENT, ATSDR   90

   Chris Portier   91

THE GENERAL   92

   Major General Eugene G. Payne, Jr.   92

THE VETERANS ADMINISTRATION   101

   Thomas J. Pamperin   101

DENY, DELAY, SICKNESS AND DEATH 104

TOXIC VAPOR INTRUSIONS DIDN'T END IN 1987! 112

EPILOGUE..121

THE MARINES' HYMN 121

JOINT BASE PEARL HARBOR-HICKAM 123

ANOTHER WATER CONTAMINATION TRAGEDY

ABOUT THE AUTHOR 144

APPENDIX A, VETERANS AFFAIRS ADMINISTRATION 146

CAMP LEJEUNE FAMILY MEMBER PROGRAM

APPENDIX B, DOCUMENTARY, SEMPER FIDELIS: ALWAYS FAITHFUL 157

APPENDIX C, NATIONAL DEFENSE AUTHORIZATION ACT FOR FISCAL YEAR 2008....................................160

APPENDIX D, CHEMICALS AT CAMP LEJEUNE (FAQS) 165

APPENDIX E, HEALTH ISSUES 169

HOW CAN BENZENE AFFECT MY HEALTH?

TRICHLOROETHYLENE (TCE)

PERCHLOROETHYLENE (PCE)

OUR IMMUNE SYSTEM

HEALTH CONCERNS AT CAMP LEJEUNE

ADVERSE BIRTH OUTCOMES STUDY RESULTS

APPENDIX F, PFAS 195

MANY MORE MILITARY BASES WITH CONTAMINATED WATER

PFAS Could Contaminate More Than 600
Military Installations (Listed)   196

MEANING OF ABBREVIATIONS 207

BIBLIOGRAPHY 208

PROLOGUE

One vision that is embedded in the minds of anyone who remembers the events surrounding the World Trade Center tragedy is that of firemen and other first responders rushing into the buildings as others were rushing out. Truly, they lived and died by a code of conduct that places the safety of others ahead of theirs.

Now take that vision and multiply it by nearly 250 years and hundreds of thousands of dead and wounded Marines. Marines, like those heroic firemen and first responders, have been putting themselves in harm's way since 1775. Their blood has been spilled on battlefields around the world and they have asked for little in return. They placed the safety of the United States ahead of theirs. They live and die by words Semper Fidelis, Always Faithful. It is written in their red blood!

The six years I served in United States Marine Corps Active Reserves were good years, at times hard both physically and mentally, but overall good. There is no question it changed me, and I know for the better. While in the service, I met some of the finest, funniest, and most decent people I have ever met. Some, I served with for many years. The officers I served under, for the most part, were smart, tough, fair and were respected by the Marines under their command.

A special thanks to some extremely thoughtful people who helped in editing this manuscript, my daughter Stacy Swimmer, my dear friend Bev Rogers, and Suzanne Hill of Carterville, GA. I recently met Suzanne Hill through a Camp Lejeune group on Facebook. Like many Marines and their families that I have met over the years she is a most giving and thoughtful person. Thank you, Gary Tisdale and Jill Steen Dilgard, my Facebook friends, for your tireless efforts to help Camp Lejeune Marines, their families and others impacted by this tragedy and providing valuable insights to this author.

This is my second book, both are non-fiction, and both were difficult to write. This book was the most difficult. The Marines are a very important and proud part of me and always will be.

Firstly, as I did the research it soon became apparent that for three months in 1965, I drank and washed in water that contained many toxic chemicals and I could very well have serious health issues because of it. Almost everyone that I remembered and had served with had died. Some suffered horribly. Several were exceptionally good friends.

Secondly, it is a black mark on the United States Marine Corps, the Department of the Navy and the Veterans Administration. That in itself is difficult for a Marine to accept. These government organizations let us down.

The book speaks for itself. Neglect and mismanagement of water systems that about one million people both drank from and washed in for over some thirty years. Then followed by years minimizing the health effects of the poisons that were found in the water and not being honest and forthright about the quantity of benzene found in the water. The Marine Corps and the Department of the Navy knew the fuel storage system had been in disrepair for years and did little to fix it. Then this was followed by years of an inept and ineffective notification process that would have alerted those of us who drank and washed in this poison. Finally, followed by years of denial and delay by the Veterans Administration to those applying for health and disability benefits. Let us not forget the lies, lies and more lies.

Marine Corps Generals when addressing the Camp Lejeune water contamination fiasco like to say that the Corps *is one big family*. Somehow, I feel their dreadful actions speak volumes and their words are meaningless.

This book will break your heart and well it should! You may think that it has to be a work of fiction, no military service or government agency could be so cruel, devious and deceitful. This is a story of one of very worst water contamination tragedies that has ever taken place in this country and how the Marine Corps spent nearly three decades poisoning the water. Then they, along with the Department of the Navy and the Veterans Administration, spent the next four decades trying to avoid responsibility for their actions.

Have they no shame?

In late 2021, two years after the book was first published, news started breaking about Joint Base Pearl Harbor-Hickam, located on Oahu, Hawaii, and water contamination issues at that base. For six months I followed this tragedy as it unfolded. It has the makings of being as serious as the Camp Lejeune catastrophe. The original manuscript has been updated with a chapter titled Joint Base Pearl Harbor-Hickam. It is added after the epilogue.

"OH, WHAT A TANGLED WEB WE WEAVE, WHEN FIRST WE PRACTICE TO DECEIVE!" (SIR WALTER SCOTT, 1808)

In late April 2020, I received a large envelope from the United States Marine Corps containing a number of documents. Included in the packet, was a press release type leaflet published by the Marine Corps long after the wells were closed in the mid 1980's and titled "Camp Lejeune Historic Drinking Water". This glossy leaflet contained several rhetorical questions and then the Marine Corps' answers. The very first question and their answer was blatantly misleading.

As you read through this chapter ask yourself a couple of questions, was the Marine Corps and the Department of the Navy deceitful in their not acknowledging the life-threatening amount of fuel (benzene) that seeped into the underground water, and would it have made a significant difference in how government agencies would have reacted to the issue if they had known about the benzene issue early on?

The question and answer.

George Swimmer

Q: When and how were the chemicals in drinking water discovered and addressed? Were there drinking water regulations for these chemicals at the time?

A: In the early 1980s, Camp Lejeune began to test drinking water for trihalomethanes (THMs) because of new regulations that had been announced by the United States Environmental Protection Agency (EPA) for those chemicals. THMs are chemicals that are created when water is treated with chlorine. While these initial tests for THMs were being conducted, other chemicals, unidentified at the time, were sometimes interfering with the results.

Through special testing of the drinking water system in 1982, the chemicals causing the interference with THM testing were identified as trichloroethylene (TCE) and tetrachloroethylene (PCE). The test results varied between drinking water samples collected at different times. Base officials were unable to immediately identify the source of the chemicals.

Beginning in 1984, as part of the environmental cleanup program, some drinking water wells were tested near potential former disposal sites. Benzene, a volatile organic compound (VOC), was found in one of the wells serving the Hadnot Point water system. When Base officials were notified of the result, the well was taken out of _service on the same day it was found to be affected,_ _and a more comprehensive well testing effort began._ When this testing identified VOCs in specific drinking water wells, the affected wells were removed from service. There were no drinking water regulations established for these chemicals at that time.

Base investigative actions revealed leaking storage tanks, industrial activities, and one off-Base dry cleaner were the sources of the contamination. Subsequent analysis found that the normal rotation of the wells and geological factors likely caused the variation of chemical levels in the drinking water. Detailed information may be found in tables published in reports by the ATSDR and the NAS/NRC. There were no drinking water regulations established for these chemicals at the time, which further complicated the Base's efforts. Federal regulations for TCE, benzene, and vinyl chloride were published in the Federal Register in 1987 and standards became effective and enforceable in 1989; Federal regulations for PCE were published in the Federal Register in 1991 and standards became effective and enforceable in 1992.

***

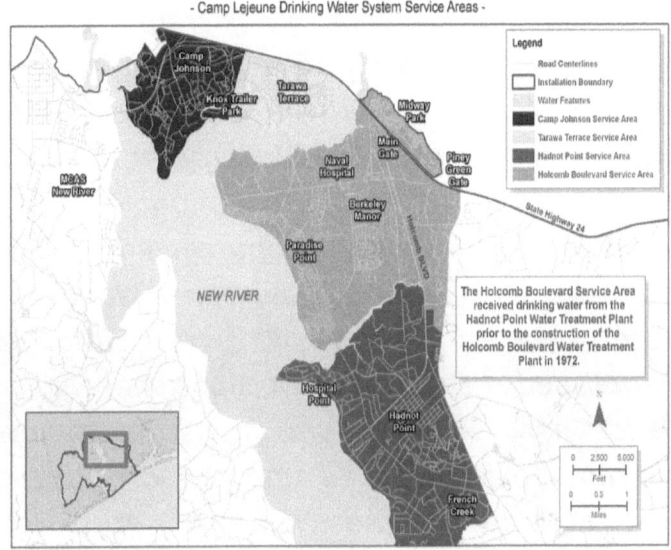

- Camp Lejeune Drinking Water System Service Areas -

The two sentences relating to the discovery of benzene were, for emphasis, underlined by this author. What I found so absolutely stunning about this admission is this, almost the instant that the benzene was found in the water the well was taken out of service and more testing was done. Certainly, the Marine Corps realized at that point in time that benzene was an extremely serious problem, even though they professed that there were no Federal regulations regarding benzene in drinking water. There had been ample information about the dangers of benzene for many years prior to the wells being closed.

Regulatory History of Benzene Exposure in the U.S.

Deadly S.N.A.F.U.

The first evidence of risk from acute or chronic effects for exposure to benzene was recognized in 1900. According to OSHA, "the benzene-leukemia link was first identified in 1897 in a report on the leukemia death of a worker occupationally exposed to benzene". Winslow recommended a 100-ppm exposure limit in 1927. Benzene's long regulatory history began in 1934, when Massachusetts established a Division of Occupational Hygiene in its Department of Labor and Industries to investigate benzene toxicity. Based upon reports by Bowditch, Hunter, Mallory, and Elkins, it set a "maximum acceptable limit" (MAC) of 75 ppm, which was soon reduced to 35 ppm. In 1946, the American Conference of Government Industrial Hygienists recommended a threshold limit value (TLV) of 100 ppm for benzene, which was lowered to 35 ppm in 1948 and 25 ppm in 1963. In 1971, OSHA adopted the voluntary industrial limit of 10 ppm, set by the American National Standards Institute (ANSI) as part of its acceptance of "national consensus standards". In that same year, the International Labor Office (ILO), a specialized agency of the United Nations, adopted ILO Convention number 136, "Convention Concerning Protection Against Hazards Arising From Benzene," which incorporated the ACGIH's standard and set an international ceiling of 25 ppm for occupational exposure. The National Institute for Occupational Safety and Health (NIOSH) issued a criteria document concerning the possible link between leukemia and benzene in 1974 (updated in 1976). A request for an emergency temporary standard (ETS) to regulate occupational exposure to benzene was filed in 1976, followed by further information from the National Academy of Sciences (NAS), which concluded that "benzene must be considered a suspect leukemogen" These conclusions, combined with the NIOSH recommendation, prompted OSHA to issue voluntary guidelines that limited the TWA to 1 ppm in 1977. OSHA then issued an ETS (which was defeated in the courts) followed by a proposed permanent standard. After extensive hearings that discussed scientific evidence in detail, OSHA issued its first final rule for the regulation of benzene in February 1978. The first final rule was challenged by labor unions and by the chemical industry, iron and steel industry, rubber manufacturers, individual companies, and the petroleum industry. The rule was vacated by the U.S. Supreme Court, in Industrial Union Department v. American Petroleum Institute (referred to as the Benzene Case) in 1980. According to OSHA, the second rulemaking was initiated in response to a petition to OSHA by labor organizations in 1984, requesting a new standard to fill the void created in the wake of the Benzene Case. OSHA's failure to provide a timely response to that petition gave rise to a petition in the federal courts, for a writ of mandamus in 1985. (If the petition before the courts *had succeeded, a writ of mandamus would have compelled OSHA to progress with the rulemaking process under the threat of contempt of court.) Instead, OSHA set forth a proposal for a rulemaking to modify the benzene standard within 14 months (1986), which defeated the labor union's petition. OSHA conducted its second benzene rulemaking in 1986. In September 1987, OSHA issued the present rule for benzene regulation. Ironically, this standard provides similar protections compared to the modified original rule, but became law without further court review.* (Feitshans 1989)

Why else would the Marine Corps react so quickly to take the well out of service when other dangerous chemicals were reported in wells years earlier and no action was taken to shut those wells down? Also, it is reasonable to believe that either at the point in time the well was taken out of service or shortly thereafter, a review of existing Camp Lejeune internal records would reflect evidence of considerable fuel leakage and spillage. The archaic and in disrepair sieve-like fuel storage facilities had been a problem for many years and was a well-known issue.

An extremely large and deadly amount of fuel, containing benzene, had seeped into at least some of the underground water supply at Camp Lejeune. Now, in a 2020 leaflet, we find out that the Marine

Corps reacted immediately. Why did a leaflet make such a self-serving admission?

That water from the deep underground water supply was sent to a filtration plant that did not remove benzene, TCE's, PCE's or any other volatile organic compounds (VOC's). The filtration process had not yet been modified to remove benzene or other VOC's from the water.

The Marine Corps answer to their rhetorical question implies that praise should be given for their immediate action in shutting down the well.

Now here is the rub. My manuscript had been written and was in final review when I received the leaflet. I decided to continue my research on the benzene issue. Again, who knew what, when did they know it, and then what did they do when they found out?

Twenty years had now passed, it was now 2004, and the Commandant of the Marine Corps General Michael W. Hagee assembled an Independent Panel that started with three people and eventually grew to five members. Their mission was to review the Camp Lejeune water supply issue from 1980 - 1985. Some Panel members had scientific or engineering backgrounds. The Chairman of the Independent Panel was former Congressman and former Naval Officer Ron Packard. The Panel proclaimed that they had reviewed over 1,600 documents, both military and civilian, and interviewed 25 people having key knowledge of the Camp Lejeune ground water issue. They took pride in the thoroughness of their investigation. The Panel issued a detailed report that indicated ten wells were closed and the primary reasons were, two wells at Tawara Terrace because of PCE, and eight wells at Hadnot Point because of TCE. Not one because of a benzene issue. The following statement is found in the Panel's report, *"The administrative record shows that several chlorinated VOCs were identified in the groundwater and tap water at Camp Lejeune during the early 1980s. Because the closure of drinking water supply wells at the base resulted from detections of TCE and PCE, the Panel addresses only these two VOCs in this report."* Benzene is a VOC and the Panel either did not consider it a serious contributing factor in the closing of any of the ten wells or, issued the disclaimer knowing far more than they wanted to include in their report. There was a passing comment relating to benzene towards the end of the very detailed report, "According to the log, Mr. Bailey informed Mr. Alexander that benzene and TCE were detected in Hadnot Point well 602." The Panel did not provide any additional detail as to the amount of benzene found in the well. The report provided considerable detail about the TCE and PCE levels of contamination. (Report 2004)

All of my research indicated that various organizations targeted to investigate the Camp Lejeune water issue; the Environmental Protection Agency Criminal Investigation Report in 2005, Government Accountability Office (GAO) whose report was issued to Congress in 2007, the National Research Council (NRC) whose report was issued 2009, and the Agency for Toxic Substances and Disease Registry (ATSDR) whose first report was originally issued in 1997 and later rescinded and then reissued after benzene became a relevant issue, were not aware of the large quantity of fuel that had leaked into the deep underground water supply. In fact, the ATSDR during their investigation had complained that it had difficulties in obtaining meaningful information from the Department of the Navy.

A Hearing held before the House Subcommittee on Oversight and Investigations of the Committee on Energy and Commerce on June 12, 2007 included many key players involved in the Camp Lejeune issue. Some of those testifying were Major General Robert Dickerson, Jr., Commanding General, Camp Lejeune, Thomas Sinks, Deputy Director, National center of Environmental Health, Agency for Toxic Substances and Disease Registry, ATSDR, accompanied by Frank Bove, Senior

Epidemiologist, ATSDR, and Morris Maslia, Environmental Engineer, Peter J. Murtha, Director, Office of Criminal Enforcement, Forensics and Training, Office of Enforcement and Compliance Assurance, U.S. Environmental Protection Agency, Marcia D. Crosse, Director, Public Health and Military Health Care Issues, U.S. Government Accountability Office, Franklin Hill, Director, Superfund Division, U.S. Environmental Protection Agency. The Hearing was lengthy and meant to be a comprehensive review of all of the issues relating to the contaminated water. It included written statements and witness testimony. The transcript filled over 400 pages that contained more than 55,000 words. A Microsoft Word search indicated that <u>TCE and PCE were mentioned about 200 times</u>. It would be fair to say that these two VOC's controlled the focus of the hearing. <u>The word "benzene" was **not** mentioned once.</u> (Transcript 2007)

Investigators, from the results shown in their reports placed little, if any, emphasis on benzene as being a significant factor in the contamination problem at Camp Lejeune.

In 2009, now some 25 years after the contaminated wells were closed and some five years after the Commandant's Report was issued, ATSDR investigators would first begin finding out that large quantities of fuel, containing benzene, had seeped into the deep underground water supply decades earlier. An ATSDR sub-contractor was inadvertently given access to a Department of the Navy database website. The investigator uncovered information about massive fuel leaks that occurred at Camp Lejeune's Hadnot Point Fuel Farm's (HPFF) storage area. The archaic storage facility had been in disrepair for years prior to the closing of the wells. For many years prior to the wells being closed the Marine Corps and the Department of the Navy knew about the fuel leakage problems. Unfortunately, investigators from government agencies and others trying to perform public health assessments did not. Also, the Marine Corps and the Navy knew Hadnot Point well number 602, from a sampling drawn in July 1984, had levels of benzene that were 380 parts per billion (ppb) which far exceeded the safety limit set by federal regulators of 5 parts per billion. <u>As time passed, the records were falsified by a Marine Corps consultant who changed records to read benzene 38 ppb and eventually again changed records to read benzene at zero ppb</u>. (B. Barrett, Lejeune water probe: Did Marine Corps hide benzene data? 2009)

In a detailed report published in January 1985 by Environmental Science and Engineering, Inc. of Gainesville, Florida under contract for the Naval Facilities Engineering Command Atlantic Division the following comment appears "**Of extreme importance is the high level of benzene (380 ug/L) detected in the sample collected from deep water supply [well] No. 602 (Well 22GW3). This benzene concentration far exceeds the 10'5 human health risk limit of 6.6 ug/L; therefore, the use of this well should be discontinued immediately.**" (Environmental Science and Engineering 1985)

"It is weird that it went from 380 to 38 and then it disappeared entirely," stated Kyla Bennett. "It does support the contention that they did it deliberately." Ms. Bennett spent 10 years as an enforcement officer for the Environmental Protection Agency before becoming an ecologist and environmental attorney. (Press 2010)

It is estimated that up to 1.1 million gallons of fuel seeped into the deep underground water at Hadnot Point over an extended period of time. The fuel was leaking for many years at a rate of 1,500 gallons a month and the Marine Corps and Navy did little to stop it. A comment in a 1988 memo from a Camp Lejeune lawyer to the base's assistant facilities manager, "It's an indefensible waste of money and a continuing potential threat of human health and the environment," wrote Staff Judge Advocate A.P. Tokarz.

At a 1988 meeting of federal, state and Lejeune officials a contractor talked about the benzene contamination and stated the water as "toxic enough for you that you don't want to touch that water."

As fuel degraded over time the levels of benzene found in the water supply increased. Tests conducted from the closed wells from June 2007 to August 2009 registered 3,490 ppb. of benzene.

The Marine Corps and the Department of the Navy failed to address the benzene issue on a timely, forthright and candid manner. The Commandant's 2004 Independent Panel Report failed to bring attention to the seriousness of the benzene issue. The Panel report concluded that the Marine Corps was not at fault. It used such reasoning as federal regulations were not in place for VOC contamination in water at the time and in the 1980's filtration of VOC's from the water at other than Camp Lejeune filtration plants was just starting to occur. The two filtration plants at Camp Lejeune had not yet been updated for VOC removals.

The Commandant's Independent Panel's final conclusion stated, **"The Panel found the Marine Corps acted responsibly, and saw no evidence of Marine Corps attempts to cover up information that indicated contamination in Camp Lejeune drinking water."**

If the Marine Corps was honest and forthright a fairly basic review of existing documents would have shown the presence of high levels of benzene in the water. Certainly, the leakage of thousands upon thousands of gallons of fuel over a period of many years would not put the Marine Corps in a good light. Now, add to that, the Marine Corps knew of the prolonged leakage and disrepair of the fuel storage facilities and did little to correct the problem. The Panel's disclaimer early on in the report eliminated almost any focus on the benzene issue. In reality, it just made a very bad situation even worse.

On September 16, 2010 the House of Representative Subcommittee on Investigations and Oversight held another extensive hearing. Finally, benzene became a centerpiece of the hearing. A Microsoft Word search of the lengthy hearing transcript indicated the word <u>"benzene" now appeared nearly 100 times.</u> From not being mentioned at a similar hearing some two years earlier it now drew the attention of everyone at the hearing.

U.S. Representative and Hearing Chairman Brad Miller's opening statement at the hearing is most powerful. He expressed the feelings of many, myself included.

PREPARED STATEMENT OF CHAIRMAN BRAD MILLER

The title of today's hearing is: "Camp Lejeune: Contamination and Compensation, Looking Back, Moving Forward." For thirty years, as many as one million Marines and their families training and living on the base at Camp LeJeune were exposed to toxic chemicals in their drinking water. Solvents such as trichloroethylene (TCE) and perchloroethylene (PCE) and by-products of fuel such as benzene leeched into the base water supply and were consumed by Marines, their wives, their children and by members of the community who worked on the base.

We will never be certain about all the adverse health consequences that come from consuming that toxic cocktail, but we can be certain that some Marines and some dependents will develop cancers that will shorten their lives. We are certain that the Marine [Corps] failed to close the wells promptly when they were informed of the presence of TCE and PCE in their water. Instead, they provided that water to their people for two more years.

The wells were shut down in the mid-1980s. For the two decades since the Marine [Corps] leadership and the Department of the Navy have denied that they have a water problem. Because "no law was broken" and the contaminated wells were, eventually, shut down, the Navy continues to deny that they bear responsibility for taking care of these veterans and their families. Children have died from rare forms of leukemia, but the Navy says they are not responsible. Marines and dependents have developed male breast cancer, but the Navy says, "not our problem". While the Department of Veterans Affairs has begun to extend benefits for cancers that they view as "more likely than not" caused by drinking the toxic water, the Navy continues to wait for scientific certainty of causation.

The Navy expresses deep concern, and waits on science to answer with certainty the question of whether the toxic chemicals they admit contaminated the water at LeJeune are responsible for any adverse health conditions. As anyone who has followed science in public health should know, there will never be scientific certainty that any particular disease in any particular person is tied to any particular exposure. Toxic chemicals and human health tends to be about probabilities, not certainties. Science will never give the Navy certainty and so long as they wait, no veteran and no family members will ever receive their due from the Navy.

The Marine Corps has recently put out a glossy booklet regarding the history of Camp Lejeune's drinking water and their response to the toxic contamination at the base. It may be their side of the story, but it is not the complete factual history of what happened to Camp Lejeune's drinking water supply, nor does it accurately portray when the Marines became aware of these known hazards, how they responded to this information or the actual public health implications of these toxic chemicals on those exposed to them.

Relying on the advice of lawyers, hiding behind science that is slow and uncertain, and spending more energy on public relations than on helping Marines and their families, the leadership of the Marine Corps and Navy appears to have qualified their sense of service and obligation by concerns about possible legal liability. They are faithful only to the point where their attorneys tell them not to admit responsibility or accept liability.

The facts are these: The U.S. Marine Corps failed to act quickly or forcefully enough in the 1980s to close down water supply wells it knew were contaminated with toxic chemicals that were endangering the health and safety of its Marines and their families on Camp Lejeune.

Deadly S.N.A.F.U.

I would like to understand why it took so long for the Marine Corps to respond because they have so far failed to provide an adequate explanation to the public, Congress or the Marines who served at Camp Lejeune and their families. I hope that U.S. Marine Corps Major General Payne can help address those issues today. For its part, the Agency for Toxic Substances and Disease Registry (ATSDR), a sister agency of the Centers for Disease Control and Prevention (CDC), produced a Public Health Assessment of human health hazards posed by Camp Lejeune's drinking water supply in 1997 that was inadequate. I am glad to see that the agency has acknowledged that inadequacy and withdrew this publication last year. The 1997 health assessment evaluated the public health impact from exposures to TCE and PCE that infiltrated the drinking water supply at Camp Lejeune up through the 1980s, but it failed to investigate and evaluate the effect of benzene contamination at the base at that time. It is critically important that ATSDR carry out its slate of promised studies as quickly as possible. These studies will not provide the certainty regarding exposure and disease that some expect, but they should help identify the range of possible cancers and other conditions that could be produced from exposure to the polluted drinking water at Camp LeJeune.

We will also hear from the Department of Veterans Affairs today. I am pleased that the VA has begun to award some Camp Lejeune veterans for illnesses they developed that the VA has found were "more likely than not" caused by exposures to toxic chemical contamination in the drinking water at Camp Lejeune. Two of our witnesses are among the half dozen awards the VA has already granted. But that leaves dependents of Marine veterans who have been harmed by these exposures, like Mike Partain, to fall through the cracks.

I introduced a bill last year called the Janey Ensminger Act that would have the VA provide health care services to both veterans and their family members who have experienced adverse health effects as a result of exposure to contaminated drinking water at Camp Lejeune. The bill is named for Janey Ensminger, a 9-year old girl who died from childhood Leukemia in 1985 after being exposed to the water at Camp Lejeune while in utero. Her father is 24-year Marine Corps veteran Jerry Ensminger who has been a tireless advocate for military families exposed to contamination at Camp Lejeune.

I believe the VA has begun to move in the right direction by awarding this small pool of veterans the compensation they need and deserve. I believe it is time that the Department of the Navy and U.S. Marine Corps stop fighting these efforts, and focus their energies on taking care of their own now and in the future. It is time that the leadership of the Navy and Marine [Corps] lived up to the motto of the Corps. They could learn from the example of Jerry Ensminger, who has been faithful always to the memory of his daughter and to all the victims of the toxic drinking water at Camp Lejeune.

20

CAMP LEJEUNE

Marine Corps Base Camp Lejeune is a 246-square-mile United States military training facility near Jacksonville, North Carolina. The base's 14 miles of beaches make it a major area for amphibious assault training, and its location between two deep-water ports allows for fast deployments. The Marine Corps is a component of the Department of the Navy.

For over three decades anyone who was stationed or lived at Marine Corps Base Camp Lejeune, North Carolina in all probability drank contaminated water, washed in it, was sickened from it, and may have eventually died from it. High levels of chemical solvents that included, trichloroethylene (TCE), perchloroethylene (PCE), methylene chloride, vinyl chloride, benzene, and toluene contaminated the water. An estimated 1,000,000 Marines, Navy, their families, workers and others drank and washed with this poison. Many more will become sick and die, the only question is when. It may take years, but it definitely will occur. (Contaminated Water Supplies at Camp Lejeune 2009)

After boot camp in Parris Island, S.C. many Marines, like myself, went to Camp Geiger for about six weeks for infantry training. Camp Geiger is considered part of Camp Lejeune and from there to main side Camp Lejeune.

For three months in 1965 I was considered stationed at Camp Lejeune. For years, Marines like myself never suspected there was a problem with the water. Many I suspect still don't. When the Marine Corps and the United States government finally acknowledged the problem, they were not forthright and honest about the seriousness of the problem and delayed for decades alerting those who spent time living or working on the base. Some of us were never notified, and those that were and filed VA claims fought tooth and nail with the Veterans Administration (VA) for benefits.

Some of the questions this book will answer; when did the Marine Corps first become aware of the contaminated water, what did they do about it and when did they do it? Also, did they knowingly delay in alerting those of us impacted? The lack of positive and direct notification continues to be a problem.

Those who were stationed, lived, worked or were conceived by someone who was at Camp Lejeune are at a higher risk of having serious health issues. Over time our immune systems will become less capable of dealing with the poisonous chemicals we drank or absorbed years earlier. Earlier testing and screenings may have led to more favorable outcomes. Lifestyle changes might have also reduced future health risks.

The water contamination problem at Camp Lejeune will be a dark chapter in the Marine Corps gallant folklore. Sadly, this is a story that must be told.

For nearly thirty years I investigated train accidents. My non-fiction book "Railroad Collisions, A Deadly Story of Mismanaged Risk" tells in detail how important it is to adequately manage risk. Time after time I would investigate an accident and knew that if just one of several contributing factors was either eliminated or mitigated the probability of the accident occurring would have been reduced. Establishing timelines, identifying contributing factors and understanding behavior patterns are critical in any accident investigation.

Camp Lejeune's water contamination tragedy occurred over decades and still continues. Along the way there have been many factors that have contributed to this tragedy. The inept and unconscionable behavior shown by the Marine Corps and the Department of the Navy is inexcusable.

Recently, I became aware of the Camp Lejeune water contamination calamity. My railroad book took many years of investigating, researching and writing. Although research is essential in any nonfiction manuscript, this book will be written and published as soon as humanly possible. Official notifications to those poisoned at Camp Lejeune have been ineffective and delayed for decades, and in many cases have never taken place. Hopefully, this book may help in that notification process.

As I did research, new issues were uncovered. The book would have begun and ended with the Camp Lejeune issue, that was, until I saw the documentary *Semper Fidelis: Always Faithful.* In the film, it was noted that 126 military bases had contaminated water problems. The film was released some eight years ago, now in 2020, the number could be over 600 U.S. military bases with contaminated water issues.

It is not unusual for a small group of passionate, strong-willed and well-meaning individuals to accomplish much. You will find such a group in the award-winning documentary *Semper Fidelis: Always Faithful.* This film not only focuses on the problems at Camp Lejeune, but it also shows us the very best of the human spirit. Thank you to this small group, those featured in the film and others, who have worked so long and so passionately to notify us of this Camp Lejeune calamity. Your energies in making this film, whether a Marine or not, and continuous efforts to make life better for others, bring truth to the Marine motto, Semper Fi.

Deadly S.N.A.F.U.

S.N.A.F.U. (situation normal all fucked up) is a term a Marine will hear often. This book is about a very deadly S.N.A.F.U. that began decades ago and still continues.

MARINES I SERVED WITH

Marine Corps Recruit Depot Parris Island, South Carolina was a miserable place to be at in the hot and humid summer of 1965, especially for a boot like myself. It was twelve weeks of intense physical conditioning, small arms weapons training, marching, marching and more marching. If my drill instructor wasn't shouting at me for screwing up, he was shouting at someone else in the platoon. Their mission was to instill discipline, that is the Marine Corps way, and it was the only way.

About the tenth week into boot camp my Platoon 143 was designated as the service platoon. Each member in the platoon was assigned a specific duty. Mine was as a guard in the mess hall. I was given a duty belt and a painted helmet liner, called a chrome dome, used to alert other recruits that I was on duty. I was instructed to make sure that recruits exiting the mess hall moved in an orderly fashion.

All of a sudden someone pushed me from behind. I turned in anger and in a split second that anger changed. It was my best friend Jim Rogers from Amundsen High School in Chicago. Jim and I played football together, were in the same club, and were constant companions. I didn't know Jim had joined the Marines. What a wonderful and special moment.

Jim died in 2016. For years he had many serious health issues. Finally, after years of being diagnosed with Barrett's Esophagus, a doctor discovered he had cancer of the kidney and performed surgery.

For nearly 60 years we were best friends. When Jim and his wife Beverly didn't show up at my daughter's October 2016 wedding, I knew something terrible must have occurred. Dan, his son called, and gave me the news of his death.

Recently, when I became more aware of the Camp Lejeune water contamination issue, I asked Jim's wife Beverly if she had ever been notified of the problem by the Marine Corps or any government agency. She had not been. I asked if she was aware that veteran health benefits would have been available for Jim. She was not.

Bev's response did not surprise me, I was also not notified.

Amundsen High School in Chicago is a couple of miles from the 2nd Battalion, 24th Marines, 4th Marine Division Reserve Unit Headquarters. Two platoons from the 2nd Battalion met at this location. Many of us either knew each other from high school or from the neighborhood. If we didn't know each other when we joined the Marine Corps, we soon became friends. We spent many years together; our obligation was six months active duty and five and half years in the active reserves, meeting one weekend a month and a yearly two-week session of training in the summer at a military base. Our wives or girlfriends also knew each other. Many of us went out socially together. Unfortunately, I have lost track of most.

***

Herb Gibson was also a high school friend. Like Jim, we played football together and were in the same club. Although I had joined the Marines some months before Herb, we were assigned to the same unit at the reserve center. He died in 2003 after having a liver transplant. He was 58 years old.

***

Dave Rogers was also a high school friend. He was Jim Rogers' cousin and had joined the reserve unit sometime before I had and in fact had talked to someone at the unit to help me with the enlistment process. Dave was an outstanding athlete, playing football at both the high school and college level. When Jim's wife Beverly recently told me that Dave had died in 2019, I was saddened but not surprised. Dave had been sick for years. About ten years before his death, I had sold Dave a large annuity, in the

$100,000 range. When we met, I knew he was struggling health wise. It was important to Dave that his former wife Barb receive the proceeds from the annuity upon his dead. Dave knew he was not insurable for life insurance at the time. Beverly told me Dave died broke spending all his money to cover his health costs. I mentioned the annuity and how important it was to him to leave it to Barb. Dave had cashed in the annuity, surely not realizing that he may have been eligible for VA health benefits.

Some 50 years ago Dave and I attended Northern Illinois University. At the time he mentioned that if I served 180 days on active duty, I would be eligible for an Illinois Veterans Grant that would pay my tuition. I mentioned that my active-duty time was considered active duty for training purposes by the VA and I am not be eligible for VA benefits. Dave said that was not the case with the Illinois Veterans Grant. He was right. I had served 182 days active duty and the Grant saved me thousands of dollars. If Dave had known, he might have been eligible for VA health and disability benefits just maybe he would not have spent his last dollar on health care costs.

***

Tom Carroll was also from the neighborhood and also in my unit at the reserve center. Tom was both one of the strongest and most decent individuals I have ever met. Tom died in 2003. His obituary did not state the cause of death or his age. Tom must have been in is late 50's or very early 60's. I just recently became aware of his death. Tom was a very special person.

***

Ron Rosario died in 2018. Ron was always fun to be around and I had the pleasure of hearing one of his many jokes or being involved in one of his many pranks for about five years. At times he had me laughing until I had tears in my eyes. Although we were not in boot camp together, we were on the same gun in the 81mm mortar platoon for many years. There was a special chemistry that was formed with Ron and almost everyone in the mortar platoon. He was a good friend, and I should have stayed in touch.

***

Roger Ludwig was in my platoon at Parris Island and was also in my reserve unit. I knew Roger fairly well in Parris Island. He died in 2008 at age 64 in a nursing home. I would suspect he had been ill for some time.

***

Les Zuziak and I became close friends at the reserve center prior to boot camp. We went through boot camp together, were in the same reserve unit for six years and hung out together for many years. Les died in 2019 from a rare form of leukemia. For years we had lost touch and I regret that. When I saw his obituary, even though many years had passed since last seeing Les, I still felt that I had lost a good friend.

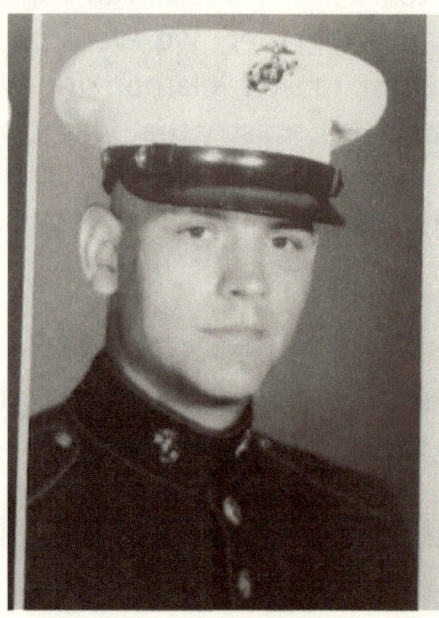

His wife Pauline was not aware of the Camp Lejeune contaminated water issue until I told her in March 2020. Les had never been notified by the Marine Corps or anyone else of the problem.

LESTER ZUZIAK

Later in the book there is a chapter "More Likely Than Not" that will address a serious question raised by Pauline Zuziak.

***

Anthony M. Kreiser was in my platoon at Parris Island and in the reserves. He died in 2007 at age 63.

***

Thomas J. Kelly was in my boot camp platoon at Parris Island. On March 3, 1970, while on duty as a Chicago Police Officer he was shot and killed. After our six months of active-duty time Tom was assigned to a reserve unit that met on the south side of Chicago and we lost touch. My unit met on the north side. Although, I did meet him once when I went to the museum and he was patrolling outside as a police officer. We talked for a few minutes and as always Tom was friendly and personable. Sadly, the next time I heard his name was when I learned of his death. Chicago Police Thomas Neustrom was shot twice when attempting to help his partner Tom Kelly.

***

For about five years William Bosak and I were together in the 81mm mortar platoon and became friends. Like Tom Kelly, he too was a Chicago Police

Officer who was shot and killed while on duty. He was killed on March 3, 1979. Chicago Police Officer Roger Van Schaik was also shot and killed in the same ambush that killed William Bosak.

***

Although the focus of this book is Camp Lejeune and the contaminated water issue, I wanted to show my thanks and respect to four Chicago Police Officers that were shot while keeping us protected. Two were Marines that I served with.

After a limited amount of computer searches for Marines I had served with, I soon realized just how serious and deadly the water contamination problem was at Camp Lejeune. Almost everyone I searched for was dead. Many, if not all, I suspect died not knowing that they may had been poisoned from drinking and washing in the contaminated water at Camp Lejeune, North Carolina.

As we grew older our immune systems became less protective and the contaminated water we drank and washed in years earlier began to take its toll.

In almost every obituary there was a reference to the time served as a Marine. Even in death it meant something to be called a Marine.

LETTER AND RESPONSES

For many years I have been an activist working to improve railroad safety. Early on, I learned how powerful a strong letter delivered to the right person can be. In late February 2020, I wrote the following letter, personalized it and mailed it to twenty-nine influential government and military leaders.

February 27, 2020

Dear XXXXX   :

Poisoned Marines need your help!

In 1965 I served about three months at Camp Lejeune, NC. As a Marine reservist I was told that I was not entitled to VA benefits.

I have lost contact with members from my Chicago based reserve unit. Two close friends died. Like myself, they did time at Camp Lejeune. Jim died in 2016 several years after being operated on for kidney cancer. Herb died in 2003 after receiving a liver transplant. Both were also friends from high school.

Deadly S.N.A.F.U.

Recently, I became aware that the water at Camp Lejeune was highly contaminated for many years, including the period I served. The Marines knew of the problem for well over thirty years. Both regular and reservists are now entitled to health and other VA benefits if they have certain diseases. The government now presumes these specific diseases were the result of this contaminated water.

Neither the Marines, nor any government agency, has ever notified me of a water problem or that I would be entitled to VA benefits. Jim's widow says her family was not notified. I believe Herb was not notified. There was no mention of it at his memorial event. Thousands of Marines either drank or washed in this poison and I believe many have not been notified.

Can you help in developing a method to officially and immediately notifying all Marines and National Guard members who served at Camp Lejeune from August 1, 1953 to December 31, 1987 of the problem and that benefits are available?

Respectfully,

George Swimmer

George Swimmer

Email: georgeswimmer1@gmail.com

***

My first response was an email received from the Veterans Administration:

Good afternoon, Mr. Swimmer.

Thank you for contacting the Department of Veterans Affairs (VA). We recorded your inquiry under Case Number XXXXXXX. If you wish to follow-up with the White House VA Hotline at 1-855-948-2311, please provide the Agent with that Case Number. This will allow us to better assist you.

The Honoring America's Veterans and Caring for Camp Lejeune Families Act of 2012, Public Law (P.L.) 112-154, was enacted on August 6, 2012, and allows for the presumption of service-connection for certain conditions affecting Veterans who served at Camp Lejeune. We regret you did not receive information about P.L. 112-154 sooner. Whenever new legislation is enacted to provide benefits for Veterans, VA works to widely publicize the event through the news, media, and other sources of public information. VA also collaborates with national and State Veterans Service Organizations (e.g., American Legion, Veterans of Foreign Wars, Disabled American Veterans, California Department of Veterans Affairs, etc.) to provide information about all benefits for Veterans and their families. General information about VA benefits, and how to apply for benefits, is available on our official website.

Developing VA Regulations

When developing regulations for administering benefits, VA must publish each proposed rule in the Federal Register to allow for comments from the public. The public comment period remains open for 60 days. Then, VA will publish the final rule, which may contain changes from the proposed rule based on the public comments received. The attached document shows the final rule for handling claims for benefits from Veterans with service at Camp Lejeune. It was published on January 13, 2017.

Disability Benefits

For general information about benefits for Veterans who served at Camp Lejeune, please see below.

To be eligible for benefits for a presumptive service-connected disability, Veterans must have served at Camp Lejeune for at least 30 days between August 1, 1953, and December 31, 1987, and later developed one of the following eight conditions:

Adult leukemia

Aplastic anemia and other myelodysplastic syndromes

Bladder cancer

Kidney cancer

Liver cancer

Multiple myeloma

Non-Hodgkin's lymphoma

Parkinson's disease

Veterans eligible for presumptive service connection include former Reservists and National Guard members who were discharged under conditions other than dishonorable.

How to Apply for Disability Benefits

There are several ways for Veterans to seek benefits:

Apply online using eBenefits. File under one of the presumed Camp Lejeune illnesses in the application. The application should include evidence of service at Camp Lejeune during the required timeframe, and medical evidence showing a diagnosis.

Please visit: https://www.ebenefits.va.gov/ebenefits/homepage

Work with a representative of an accredited Veterans Service Organization, or an agent. Find one at: https://www.va.gov/ogc/apps/accreditation/index.asp

Go to a VA regional office and get assistance from a VA employee. Find the nearest

*office
at: https://www.va.gov/directory/guide/division.
asp?dnum=3*

For more information about disability benefits, you can use the following link.

https://www.benefits.va.gov/COMPENSATION/claims-postservice-exposures-camp-lejeune-water.asp

Health Care Benefits

For general information about VA health care benefits, including family member health care reimbursement, you can use the link shown below.

https://www.publichealth.va.gov/exposures/camp-lejeune/

I hope you find this information helpful. Thank you for your service to our great nation.

Deadly S.N.A.F.U.

Veteran Benefits Administration

Department of Veterans Affairs

***

The VA's notification process is inadequate. Many, if not most veterans, whether regulars or reservists do not belong to the organizations mentioned. To count on the news media to deliver an important and meaningful message and for the VA to assume that all the people impacted either heard the message or understood the seriousness of it is a misguided approach. Would a veteran not in need of health benefits search the VA website for health benefit issues? A reservist would have no reason to search it even if in need of health benefits. It was clearly stated upon discharge our active duty was for training and did not qualify for VA benefits.

***

A letter dated March 27, 2020 was received from A. M. Niebel, Colonel, USMC, Chief of Staff, Marine

Corps Installations Command was thoughtful and detailed. It was sent on behalf Secretary of Defense Esper. In it the Colonel indicated that his staff added my name to a notification data, and I would begin receiving health study and VA benefit information.

The Colonel went on to state that since the establishment of the notification database in 2007 the Marine Corps has registered over 270,000 unique names and collected more than 130,000 email addresses that are utilized for notification and outreach. Other forms of media such as social media and newspapers were used to encourage others who may have drank or washed in the contaminated water to register.

***

The following testimony reflects just how inept the Marine Corps leadership was in their notification process.

June 12, 2007 Hearing, House of Representatives Subcommittee on Oversight and Investigations

Congressman Stupak to General Dickerson. General Dickerson was Commanding

Deadly S.N.A.F.U.

Officer at Camp Lejeune:

And General Dickerson, let me ask you this. Why has DoD not notified those residents at Camp Lejeune who were there during the time these wells were in use, that they may have been exposed to TCE or PCE?

General DICKERSON. *Sir, there have been numerous communications from the commanding general at the time, from Headquarters Marine Corps, through media surveys, contacted over 3,500 media outlets, whether that be weekly publications, daily publications.*

Mr. STUPAK. *I realize that. The people who were there, you can't tell me the Marine Corps doesn't know who was at Camp Lejeune from 1965 to 2007.*

General DICKERSON. *We could probably get the data who was stationed at Camp Lejeune. Would it be 100 percent complete? I'm not sure. We've made every attempt to get the information out and work with ATSDR to make sure——*

Mr. STUPAK. *Right. I mean military—don't you think you have a responsibility to let these people know they may have been exposed?*

General DICKERSON. *Yes, sir.*

Mr. STUPAK. *Why don't you do it?* (Transcript 2007)

***

Later at the same hearing.

Congressman W_{ALDEN}. *I am sorry to interrupt you. I am going to run out of time here. I want to go to one other point you said, because you talked about, you got a letter notifying you of potential health risks from Camp Lejeune.*

General D_{ICKERSON}. *Yes, sir.*

Mr. W_{ALDEN}. *Do you know how many of those letters went out?*

General D_{ICKERSON}. *It was my information and knowledge that everybody living on the base got one of those official letters. Now whether they were received or not I cannot testify to this committee.*

Mr. W_{ALDEN}. *I understand, but this is everybody living on the base at the time you were living on the base?*

General D_{ICKERSON}. *Yes, sir.*

Mr. W_{ALDEN}. *Not that they tracked down those who had lived on the base.*

General D_{ICKERSON}. *No, sir, at that point in time, from the commanding general, it was those who were living on the base.* (Transcript 2007)

***

The VA in 2010 stated the Marine Corps had the names of one million Marines who were stationed at Camp Lejeune during the contaminated water timeframe. Although the Colonel's information didn't indicate exactly how many Marines were notified it seems to be far less than the total population impacted. It took forty years after the Marine Corps first became aware of the contaminated water for my name to be added to a notification database and that only occurred after action on my part. Since the notification database was established in 2007 the Marine Corps in 2020 should have been able to know the total number of Marines at Camp Lejeune during the period specified, how many had died, and how many of those who were still living were notified and had responded. The Colonel's March 27, 2020 letter did not address these points. It also did not answer a key question, were the Active Reserves ever notified directly?

During my forty-five years as a Certified Public Accountant, I performed many audits of a company's financial statements. One method of confirming transactions and balances was to send out positive confirmations. The seriousness of the water contamination problem leads me to believe that a positive confirmation may very well have been the most logical approach. Simply put, each person stationed at Camp Lejeune during August 1, 1953 to December 31, 1987 is notified through mail, that person is then requested to acknowledge receipt of the notification letter by returning through prepaid postage a notification receipt. Those not responding are accounted for in any one of a number of ways, Social Security, Internal Revenue Service (IRS), FBI, etc., all having databases that would have been helpful in locating addresses and determining whether a person was still living.

Three high quality databases could have been formed, those who responded, those who had died, and those for whom additional research is required.

In fact, Commander James Watters indicated in testimony before the Subcommittee on Investigations and Oversight held on September 16, 2010 that he was first notified in a letter from General Payne of the contaminated water issue. The letter was enclosed in an IRS envelope and received around July 2008. Commander Watters had been notified by his doctor in November 2007 that he had renal cell carcinoma, stage 3, almost stage 4. In January 2008 he was told by his doctor that he had about a year to live. (Hearing Serial # 111-108 2010)

With a meaningful effort a high percentage of the Marines would have been notified in a relatively short period of time. Why delay this notification for decades, and in many cases not at all?

Life insurance companies would have been able to give the Marine Corps insights on how to best accomplish the notification process. They have departments setup to search for beneficiaries of policies when death benefits have not yet been claimed.

The four military Services spent over $600 million on recruiting advertising in 2007. This represents a 150 percent increase since the 1999 fiscal year (FY). (Dertouzos 2009)

Surely, a better effort should have been made to notify Marines, Sailors, dependents, and workers.

MORE LIKELY THAN NOT

A survey taken by ATSDR of 12,598 children born at the base between 1968 and 1985 showed an increased risk of childhood cancers and birth defects, such as spina bifida. The survey began in 1968 because that was the first year that computerized birth certificates became available. (Twedell 2013)

More than 1,000 babies were stillborn or died at infancy on the base from 1947 to 1987, according to an exhaustive survey of death certificates filed with the county.

In an article written in 2012 titled "Camp Lejeune water contamination victim speaks out" William McMurray, Jr., 29 years old, tells of his various health issues; spina bifida, Asperger's syndrome, Tourette's Bipolar disorder, Organic brain dysfunction, and more. For the first 20 years of his life doctors couldn't explain why he had all these ailments. That was until they learned of Lejeune's water contamination.

"I spent so long not knowing why I am the way I am. When they finally found the conditions and why I was like this I was so ticked." McMurray stated.

From Michael Pertain's testimony at a Congressional hearing "You have male breast cancer" were the words which greeted me and my wife on our 18th wedding anniversary. My name is Michael Partain and I am the son and grandson of United States Marine Corps officers. My parents were stationed aboard Marine Corps Base Camp Lejeune shortly after my father graduated from the United States Naval Academy. I was conceived, carried and then born at the base Naval Hospital during the drinking water contamination period at Camp Lejeune.

Three years ago, I was diagnosed with male breast cancer at the age of 39. In fact, I am one of 64 men who share the unique commonality of male breast cancer and exposure to the contaminated water aboard Camp Lejeune. There is no history of the disease in my family, and I have tested negative for the hereditary breast cancer markers BRCA1 and BRCA2. I do not drink nor do I smoke." (Hearing Serial # 111-108 2010)

The large number of stillborn births and those who died at infancy is significant evidence that something was occurring at conception or during prenatal development that was causing a serious problem. And the presumption is that this serious problem was caused by the contaminated water. There is also ample evidence that children born on the base faced a wide range of diseases and health issues. Also, many health issues appeared later in their lives. The examples above are just two of many.

It has always been believed that stillborn births and children with birth defects were a result of the mother being on the base. (Kay 2012)

It seems that the paternal parent was not considered as a factor at conception or during prenatal development for any of the health issues that put the fetus at risk.

This chapter is meant to put a red flag on that train of thought.

My book was first published in paperback in late June 2020 and Pauline Zuziak, Lester's widow, purchased the first paperback copy. Within a couple of days after purchasing it I received the following note from her.

George, I just received your book this morning and was just wondering if anything could be passed down to our kids? Our oldest son has or had Barrett's (mentioned by your friend Beverly). Not sure if he still has Barrett's, but the doctor told him about this. I don't want to scare him about this. Have you heard of any offspring's having problems?

Also, our middle son was diagnosed with a brain tumor when he as 10, it was cancer but a very slow growing one and took 10 years to cause a problem. A germinoma tumor. Then in 2007 this same son suffered a massive stroke caused by a rare myxoma tumor in his heart. It's got me wondering if Les passed something on to our sons. Our third son is healthy and just overworked. What do you think?

Pauline's comment took me by surprise and frankly was one of those "oh my God" reactions. The son of someone else I had also served with at Camp Lejeune was diagnosed with Type 1 diabetes at an early age.

In both situations the fathers, prior to the conception of their children, had not been at Lejeune for years and the mothers had never been on the base. In both, the fathers died of one of the illnesses that the VA had made the presumption had been connected to drinking and washing in the contaminated water. The illnesses of the fathers appeared long after the children were born.

Until now, my investigation into the Camp Lejeune contaminated water tragedy had revealed that the diseases associated with the newborn, even when the diseases appeared in later years, were only with those newborns conceived on the base.

A series of facts will support the argument that there is a more likely, than not, probability that children whose fathers who had been stationed at Lejeune but were born years after their fathers had been on the base, and the mothers having never been on the base, have an increased likelihood of acquiring diseases associated with the contaminated water.

We know that for many who had served at Camp Lejeune the diseases appeared later in their lives. Between January 2011 and June 2019, 84,000 claims were filed for benefits with the VA that related to the Camp Lejeune contaminated water. The last well was closed in 1985 and the water contamination existed for many years prior to the wells being closed. (Faith Abubey 2019)

This fact suggests several things. Many Marines had children prior to filing for VA claims. Also, the passage of time, in some cases about sixty years, would suggest many Marines, their wives and dependents may have died prior to 2011 of water contaminated type diseases and VA claims were never filed. It would also suggest that additional claims are to be filed by Camp Lejeune veterans as time passes. Also, some veterans, like myself, who are on Medicare or have good private insurance coverage would not seek VA health care benefits.

The numbers of children born to veterans who at one time in their lives drank and washed in Camp Lejeune's contaminated water would be staggering.

There are a number of scientific studies that now lead one to believe that the biological consequences of environmental exposures in the father's life before conception might affect his unborn child.

In an article titled "Chips off the Old Block: How a Father's Preconception Exposures Might Affect the Health of His Children" by author Charles W. Schmidt and published in February 2018 leads the reader in the direction that the father's preconception environmental exposures can lead to health problems for the child. Author Schmidt uses a number of sources to support his argument.

"We've been hyper focused on how the mother's environment shapes health of a developing kid while ignoring the other half of the equation. But the father's preconception exposures matter, too." Says Richard Pilsner, an associate professor in the School of Public Health, University of Massachusetts.

A study in 1974 suggested higher rates of cancer in children whose fathers were exposed to hydrocarbons on the job. Other studies suggest a connection between a father's diet and his descendants' health.

There are studies with mice that also lead us in the direction. Tracy Bale, a professor at the University of Maryland School of Medicine stated after a 2013 study with mice "What that's telling us is that mild changes to a dad's environment reprogram DNA and shift brain development in the offspring. For now, we just want to understand what's happening to the sperm and how these changes get passed down to subsequent generations." (Schmidt 2018)

A highly scientific review article "Influence of paternal preconception exposures on their offspring: published in May 2016, through epigenetics to phenotype" written by Georgetown University Medical Center, Georgetown University Special Master's Program in Physiology concluded that hazardous environmental exposures during the lifetime of the father can affect not only his immediate offspring but future generations as well. They added that future research should address deficiencies in current literature.

It should also be noted that alcohol consumption during the lifetime of the father can lead to a Fetal Alcohol Spectrum Disorders (FASD), which includes Fetal Alcohol Syndrome (FAS), in the offspring. This can be true even if the mother is a non-alcohol drinker.

(Jonathan Day 2016)

In a 2014 article "Fathers drinking: Also responsible for fetal disorders" the authors indicated that groundbreaking new research revealed that <u>until 2014</u> fathers were not linked to FAS, but groundbreaking new research indicated that the father's preconception alcohol consumption could lead to FASD disorders in the newborn. (Francis 2014)

About ten years prior to the 2014 article, I was a member of the Illinois Task Force on FASD. The focus of the task force was to better alert women to the dangers of drinking alcohol during conception and prenatal development. Included in the group were medical experts who specialized in treating children with FASD. I am not such an expert and was a non-professional citizen advocate member who at the time was a foster caregiver. The information we touted had a serious flaw in that it implied, and implied maybe be too gentle of a word, that as long as the mother did not drink alcohol during conception or during the prenatal time frame the child would not suffer from FASD issues. Now, many years later research produced new data that indicated differently.

Scientific data not only changes over time but often takes decades to accumulate.

The last scientific article I will reference in this chapter was written by Anne C. Ferguson-Smith and Mary-Elizabeth Patti and titled "You Are What Your Dad Ate" the authors discuss research studies using rats. The study explained the results that occurred when a controlled population of male rats were fed various diets and the impact it had on their offspring.

In conclusion the article stated, "Regardless, these experimental models of metabolic disease tell us that the environmental burden on offspring phenotype is not only just maternal territory: the father's nutritional and metabolic status certainly merits our attention, too, if we are to optimize health of his children and grandchildren." (Anne C. Fergusion-Smith 2011)

Shortly after reading the article I emailed some medical research investigators the following message:

This is a crazy story. I write a book about contaminated water at Marine Base Camp Lejeune. The widow of my best friend describes the health issues her husband went through, Barrett's Esophagus and kidney cancer. Her husband and I served together at Lejeune. The first paperback copy is sold to the widow of another friend I served with. Her children, now adults, have some serious health issues including Barrett's Esophagus. She wants to know if there could be a connection. She had never been on the base and the children were conceived long after her husband had been on the base. Her husband died of a rare form of leukemia long after the children were born. There is more to the story, my best friend's son has Type 1 Diabetes that he developed at an early age but long after my friend was out of the service. His wife was never on the base. There is another item to note, one million Marines and their families drank and washed in the water over about 30 years. The question is, is it more reasonable than not to believe there is a connection between the contaminated water the fathers drank and washed in and the health issues of their children that appeared years after their fathers were at the base?

Thank you, George Swimmer

One note that I received back stated that there is no data available currently to make or exclude a connection and more work is needed.

Unfortunately, the consequences of waiting for more data to accumulate is far too dangerous and not a very good way to manage risk.

It is my opinion that it is more likely than not to believe that certain diseases connected to the contaminated water that male Marines, and other

males, drank and washed in at Camp Lejeune during preconception can be passed on at conception, even if conception takes place many years after direct exposure by the father to the contaminated water!

These diseases may appear in the offspring many years after their birth, with the father not showing any disease symptoms and the mother never being directly exposed to the contaminated water at Camp Lejeune.

Some thoughts that may help in reducing risk are lifestyle changes, additional medical screenings, being more in tune to changes in your body, etc.

Does this scare of me? Sure, it does! I have three children!

Bev Rogers, the widow of my best friend Jim, when editing this chapter emailed me that she had a stillborn child in 1974. Bev had never been at Lejeune. Jim, Les Zuziak and I were discharged in 1971. The wells were not capped until many years later.

My Facebook post in July 2020 on the "The Few, The Proud, The Forgotten", a group consisting of Marine/Navy veterans who served at Camp Lejeune and their families, brought a number of comments. Sadly, many children born long after their fathers were stationed at Lejeune have serious health issues.

Deadly S.N.A.F.U.

A sampling of just some of the many comments received follows. Each person gave this author permission to reprint their comment.

Michelle Birkenstock commented,

My Dad was there 1953-1956. I was born twenty years after his discharge. He passed last year from Multiple Myeloma. I have Multiple Sclerosis. My oldest son was born with a bone defect. The contamination alters DNA. We have three generations effected by the poisoning, pray it's not 4th, 5th

Kathleen McKenzie commented,

My dad was stationed at Lejeune from '77-'79 before my sisters and I were born. We then lived there from '90-'91. My sister was diagnosed with a meningioma brain tumor in March of 2019, and I was diagnosed with uterine cancer 3 months later, and had to have a hysterectomy. We've looked into VA benefits, but were told we had to live at CL between '53-'87.

Jill Steen Dilgard commented,

My Dad was at Camp Geiger from 1952-1955. None of us kids were born there and my Mom was never there. Three of my siblings have heart issues, 1 has what they call a smoldering leukemia, another one has a slow growing blood cancer and had uterine cancer, 3 have had problems with their teeth, I have a blood disorder, have battled iron deficiency anemia on and off my whole life, IGE deficient, born with a partial mal-rotation, and had renal tubular acidosis. My Dad was the youngest of 9 kids and my Mom was the youngest of 4 kids. None of the above illnesses run on either side of the family. Both of my children have numerous health issues. My Dad passed from bladder cancer that metastasized to his bones.

He also had prostate cancer, severe peripheral neuropathy (not diabetic), his teeth crumbled and fell out, skin issues, renal toxicity, stage 3 renal insufficiency, heart issues, and on and on. (Author's note, Camp Geiger is a part of Camp Lejeune.)

Joe Aun

commented, https://www.facebook.com/joe.aun.31?__cft__%5b0%5d=AZUFN4JPIzT25JRU4qX23OTBYWJvl7eOPrEqb6SizdiZgYHnBOqd8GxO7KAtreGkv28DfKh5apnTjD7yUg3APQxp4HrMlpzIPyzCsu1b3cJwfyDfEQp67hjpQLWSfhoT4V_0n3l_cX-DvyDUsDZZWhRtYQNX19o5NGdKocthKs5loJqX_zq0fzXOM82g5uTTf4s&__tn__=R%5d-R

76-78 my daughter was conceived 4 yrs after I got out. She, at age 22 out of the blue is diagnosed with "a rare and primitive Leukemia". Suffered 4 1/2

yrs. until she succumbed. I call it MURDER! THEY KNEW THE WATER WAS TOXIC, "WATER IS WATER, MY MARINES NEED WATER" one CG said when he was told of the levels of contaminates. I've got weird skin sores, random bone/ muscle pain.

Joe Aun and I spoke on the phone for almost two hours. He is a passionate, very knowledgeable and a long-time advocate. A quick overview of our conversation. His notification from the Marine Corps came in 2008 but was a questionnaire that **did not** mention the contaminated water. In fact, he thought it had something to do with his time stationed at Camp Pendleton. He found out about the water contamination issue years later when watching an excerpt of a documentary on TV. He stated that he is very much into social media and that from visiting the Camp Lejeune issue websites he has observed many comments regarding children that were born long after their fathers had served at Camp Lejeune and the children have serious health issues similar to those presumed by the VA for veterans who served there. He stated that his daughter's oncologist indicated that there very well may have been a connection between his time at Camp Lejeune and his daughter's leukemia. He mentioned that the Marine Corps was warned as early as the 1950's by the State of North Carolina about contamination issues. He also mentioned the Yale Project, which I had heard of in passing but had not researched. Since the conversation I have researched and address the Yale Project in a later chapter.

Jon Ehrhard commented,

We were on Air Station New River and went to school on Lejeune 71-73,

My brother died of 3 cancers at 46 years old in 2008,

My mom died of 2 cancers at 68 in 2005,

I lost a kidney to cancer in 2013.

(Author's note, Marine Corps Air Station New River is located about 13 miles from Camp Lejeune. It is a much smaller facility than Camp Lejeune and I would suspect many families living at New River drove their children to school at Lejeune, used Lejeune's medical facilities, the PX, etc. VA benefits have been extended to Marines/Navy that were stationed at New River as if they had served at Camp Lejeune.)

Bridget Stull commented,

My father who passed away at 55 was there in 70-72. Both my brother and I were born premature at different places. I have had cancer 2x and am being tested for ALL. I also have Hashemites disease, and several other medical issues. My oldest daughter was born with 2 rare genetic diseases Tuberous Sclerosis Complex (doesn't have DNA to block any tumor type) and Hypo Plastic Left Heart syndrome, she also has epilepsy and autism among an arm length of medical complications. My youngest born 3 yrs later had single artery umbilical cord, was born with underdeveloped nervous system, has several auto immune disorders.

I was told there is nothing to be done since my father died years ago.

TIMELINE

Two water systems at Camp Lejeune, Tarawa Terrace and Hadnot Point that were found to be contaminated with TCE and PCE. As the tragedy unfolds it was later determined that substantial amounts of fuel, containing benzene, had also leaked into the groundwater. The water from these wells supplied drinking and washing water to most of Camp Lejeune's population; to both residential and non-residential areas including barracks, schools, the hospital and recreational and indoor training pools such as the Hadnot Point swimming pools from 1950 to 1985. (Registry, Camp Lejeune, North Carolina Jan 2017, updated)

The water was obtained through wells from a freshwater aquifer system located about 180 feet underground and was then pumped into a water treatment plant. The water from various wells was combined and then treated through several processes to remove minerals and soften the water. It did not remove the toxic chemicals that had seeped into the freshwater aquifer system. The water was then stored in reservoirs and used as needed.

<u>1953 and for over thirty years</u>: ABC One-Hour Cleaners, an off-base cleaner, as a result of spills and

improper disposal practices contaminated groundwater serving the Tarawa system with PCE. The contamination of the Hadnot Point water supply was more complex and involved multiple contaminates. The primary contaminates found in Hadnot Point water system when monitoring began was TCE. The multiple sources of contamination included on base spills, and leaks from underground storage tanks, and leaks from drums located at dumps and storage lots. (Contaminated Water Supplies at Camp Lejeune 2009)

1963 The Department of the Navy recommended the regulation of many of the worst chemicals found in the water according to 1963's Manual of Naval Preventive Medicine. (Kay 2012)

1970s The Environmental Protection Agency (EPA) called Lejeune a major polluter. (W. R. Levesque 2009)

1974 A regulation on the books at Camp Lejeune shows that the Marine Corps knew the danger organic solvents posed. (W. R. Levesque 2009)

1979 *The Hadnot Point Fuel Farm (HPFF) was constructed on the Southeast corner of Holcomb Blvd and Ash Street sometime in 1941. The fuel farm was comprised of fourteen fuel tanks buried in the ground and one large 600,000-gallon tank located above ground. The fuel farm was located in* *what is now known as the Hadnot Point Industrial area and within 1,200 feet from potable water well HP–602 which was also constructed in 1941. The first documented fuel leak at the HPFF occurred in 1979 when an estimated 20,000 to 30,000 gallons of fuel leaked from an underground valve. A condition survey for the HPFF was scheduled the following year and other problems were found at the HPFF. The LantDiv engineer concluded that because of age, failure to clean the tanks, and lack of maintenance, there had been a general condition of corrosion and deterioration of the tanks and connecting pipelines. Many of the interconnecting valves and flanges could not be inspected because they were buried and/or could not be located. The engineer recommended replacing the connecting piping, the inspection of all of the tanks for leaks and repair existing leaks. The Condition Survey was followed in 1981 with a Military Construction Data project number LE201M to repair the HPFF facilities and $537,200 was then allocated to clean and repair the petroleum tanks. By March of 1983, Navy and Marine Corps officials determined that piece meal rehabilitation of the HPFF was not cost effective and in 1985, the recommendation was made to replace the HPFF with a new facility. The fuel farm was finally replaced in 1990.* (Hearing Serial # 111-108 2010)

Deadly S.N.A.F.U.

October 31, 1980: *Documents show that the first warnings about Camp Lejeune came that year, when an Army laboratory chief began scrawling notes about chemicals that were showing up in the routine water tests.*

The lab chief, William Neal Jr., who was working for the U.S. Army Environmental Hygiene Agency, tested the water at Hadnot Point, an area with wells serving the base hospital, some barracks and officers' housing, and close to a massive underground fuel tank storage farm.

On Oct. 31, 1980: At the bottom of a one-page table of testing results, the lab chief wrote: "Water is highly contaminated with low molecular weight halogenated hydrocarbons," chemical compounds that can include many industrial organic compounds. (B. Barrett, Warnings about Lejeune's tainted water went unheeded for years 2010)

April 1982: *A Raleigh, N.C.-based contractor was hired to conduct the same routine tests for trihalomethanes, the chlorine byproducts, again at Hadnot Point and the housing community of Tarawa Terrace.*

Mike Hargett, a co-owner of Grainger Laboratories, could not do the tests he wanted to do. Organic solvents were interfering with his readings.

They were the same poisons that the Army laboratory chief had warned about.

Alarmed, Hargett began issuing repeated warnings to base officials that the wells appeared to be pumping out contaminated water.

No such standards yet existed for drinking water, but the EPA had made it clear that the chemicals posed a threat.

Hargett first picked up the phone in his Raleigh office on May 6, 1982, and called Lejeune's base chemist, Elizabeth Betz, according to documents. He told her about the TCE and the PCE.

"If that water had been the effluent of a wastewater treatment plant, that plant would have been in violation and fined," Hargett stated. (B. Barrett, Warnings about Lejeune's tainted water went unheeded for years, 2010)

<u>1983</u>: *In the spring of 1983, the Marines gave the EPA a report required in preparation for the new Superfund law on cleaning up significant hazardous-waste sites at Camp Lejeune. The report said that no sites on base "pose an immediate threat to human health."* (B. Barrett, Warnings about Lejeune's tainted water unheeded for years, 2010)

<u>1984</u>: The contaminated well was shut down in November 1984, four months after the benzene was first discovered in well #602 in July 1984.

<u>November 1984-May 1985:</u> The wells in both systems closed some four plus years after first warnings went out.

<u>1985</u> **Despite these anomalous reading, closed wells were periodically turned back on throughout 1985 to ease temporary water shortages**. In April 1985, Major General L. H. Buehl told residents of Tarawa Terrace, a nearby residential area, that the wells had been shut down strictly as a precaution based on "minute" chemical readings. <u>The affected wells were closed for good only in 1987.</u>

General Buehl died on October 5, 1988 at age 56 from a stroke. (Sarvana 2009)

<u>November 1985</u>: In a meeting which took place at the base in November of 1985, Robert Alexander told the EPA that their contractor's report was in error and resisted the idea of placing the base on the NPL. Somehow or another, the EPA walked away with the idea that no contamination was detected in treated potable water at the Hadnot Point WTP. Two weeks after this meeting, the treated water at the Hadnot Point WTP was sampled and found to contain benzene in the extreme amount of 2,500 ppb. (Hearing before Subcommittee on Investigations and

Oversight, Serial #111-108 2010) Environmental Protection Agency (EPA)

<u>1987</u> Wells that had been reopened because of water shortage are finally closed again.

<u>February 1988</u>: Question and answer press release issued by a Colonel who was Camp Lejeune's Assistant Chief of Staff, Facilities:

``Q. *Is my health or the health of my family in any danger?*

A. *No it's not. All the wells which we get our raw water out of are continually tested and the wells that were identified as being contaminated have been closed off.*''

``Q. *What about prior to 1983?*

A. *At that time we were not aware of any of these particular compounds that might have been in the ground water and we have no information that anyone's health was in any danger at that time.*''

<u>October 1989</u>: Camp Lejeune officially placed onto the National Priorities List (NPL) or Superfund List.

<u>1994</u> As early as 1994 the ATSDR began writing to the Marine Corps that they were not receiving vital

records regarding the full extent of the toxic contamination at Camp Lejeune. In 2005 the ATSDR informed the Government Accountability Office (GAO) there were a "substantial number of additional documents that had not been previously provided by Camp Lejeune officials." (Hearing Serial # 111-108 2010)

<u>2004</u> Commandant of the Marine Corps Independent Panel's Report found the Marine Corps acted responsibly and made no attempt to cover up information.

<u>2007</u>: USMC launched notification and registration campaign for former residents to sign up for more information by telephone or internet. (Water n.d.)

The notification began about 25 years after the Marine Corps was first alerted to the contaminated water issue. Many of the Marines I had served with were either dead or sick by 2007. I suspect most, if not all, like myself were never notified by the Marine Corps.

<u>2008 Notifications Required</u>: Congress requires Navy/Marine Corps to notify Marines of contaminates in the Camp Lejeune water. It is now 2020 and I was not directly notified and question whether any Marine Corps reservists were directly

notified. (National Defense Authorization Act of Fiscal Year 2008 n.d.)

2009, The National Research Council published a detailed manuscript *Contaminated Water Supplies at Camp Lejeune: Assessing Potential Health Effects Nation Research Council:* (Contaminated Water Supplies at Camp Lejeune 2009) The manuscript omitted benzene as one of the significant contaminates found in the Camp Lejeune water. The report drew some peer criticism in that it did not directly connect the contaminated water to the many health issues it caused.

2009: Documents uncovered in 2009 indicated that potentially as much as 1.1 million gallons of fuel, containing benzene, leaked from underground storage tanks, that had been neglected and in disrepair on the base during the period from August 1, 1953 through December 31, 1987. Benzene is a fuel solvent known to cause cancer in humans. (F. O. Barrett 2012)

September 16, 2010 Hearing Before the Subcommittee on Investigations and Oversight, Committee of Science and Technology, House of Representative

"U.S. Marine Corps (USMC). For thirty years, Marines and their dependents serving at Camp Lejeune were exposed to toxic chemicals in their drinking water. It took the USMC more than four years to shut down drinking water wells they knew to extent of contamination at Camp Lejeune. In the past, ATSDR has struggled to obtain complete cooperation and support from the Navy in providing them with records necessary to conduct accurate and comprehensive public health assessments of Camp Lejeune's toxic hazards. The U.S. Marine Corps continue to view past environmental contamination at Camp Lejeune as a public relations battle rather than a public health hazard. In July 2010, for instance, they released a glossy booklet on Camp Lejeune's Historic Drinking Water which excludes critical information and misrepresents scientific conclusions about the health impact of past toxic exposures on Camp Lejeune residents."

Hadnot Point water served Main side which included the base barracks, the Naval Hospital, and with that thousands of Marines, Sailors and their families. (ATSDR)

April 2011: Award winning documentary Semper Fidelis: Always Faithful is released.

August 2012: President Obama signs into law the Honoring America's Veteran and Caring for Camp Lejeune Families Act of 2012 also known as the Janey Ensminger Act. Among those in attendance at the signing ceremony were Jerry Ensminger, Janey's father, and Mike Partain. The law is to provide health care to thousands of sick Marine veterans and their families who were exposed to contaminated water at Camp Lejeune.

Retired Marine Jerry Ensminger and cancer survivor Mike Partain stood looking over the president's shoulder as he, with the swipe of his pen, vindicated all their late nights of poring over undisclosed documents, cross-country trips to seek out other victims, and countless battles with Marine Corps officials who, they say, continue to ignore their pleas.

"Sadly, this act alone will not bring back those we've lost, including [Janey] Ensminger," Obama said before signing the bill, named partly after Ensminger's daughter, "but it will honor their memory by making a real difference for those who are still suffering."

Janey Ensminger was just 9 years old when she died in 1985 of a rare form of leukemia. Her father spent years trying to make sense of her painful death. *But in 1997, he saw a news report about contaminated water at Camp Lejeune. Janey Ensminger was conceived at the base in the 1970s and diagnosed with leukemia in 1983.*

Partain, who was born on the base, already had been diagnosed with male breast cancer when he learned of Ensminger's efforts. A claims adjustor for

State Farm Insurance, Partain figured his investigative skills would be helpful to their mutual cause.

Their combined efforts eventually led to the passage of a bill, introduced by Sen. Richard Burr, R-N.C., that would provide health care for people who lived or worked at the base... (F. O. Barrett 2012)

<u>March 2017</u>: Former services member exposed to contaminated water at Camp Lejeune, under a new federal rule can now apply for disability benefits. The benefits are expected to cost more than $2 billion over the next five years. As many as one million veterans served at Camp Lejeune during the period specified in the rule. (III 2017)

<u>April 2018 released "Morbidity Study of Former Marines, Employees, and Dependents Potentially Exposed to Contaminated Drinking Water at U.S. Marine Corps Base Camp Lejeune."</u>

For cumulative exposures to TCE and PCE in internal analyses, the morbidity study found that contaminated drinking water at Camp Lejeune was associated with increased risk in both Marines and civilian employees for bladder cancer, kidney cancer, and kidney disease and that these results were formed by evidence from other studies. (Registry, Morbidity Study of Former Marines, Employees, and Dependents Potentially Exposed to Contaminated

Drinking Water at U.S. Marine Corps Base Camp Lejeune April 2018)

The above Morbidity Study did not include Marines and Navy personnel who served prior to April 1975 or civilians who served prior October 1972. It is estimated 1,000,000 persons either drank or washed in the contaminated water between August 1, 1953 and December 31, 1987. The Morbidity Study was sent to less than 25% of those who served during that time period and had a response rate of about 30%. It would be reasonable to believe that as the population of those who had either served, lived or worked at Camp Lejeune during some 34 years between August 1, 1953 and December 31, 1987 aged their immunity systems lost its ability to combat many of the diseases associated with the contaminated water. A more in-depth survey would have would have reflected more dire results.

January 2019:   The Secretary of the Navy announces that civil lawsuits arising from the Camp Lejeune water contamination from 1953 to 1987 will be denied by the Navy. At the time of the announcement there were about 4,400 claims that sought about $963 billion in damages. (Copp 2019) See Chapter "Deny, Delay, Sickness and Death"

September 2019: Investigative report by NBC Atlanta affiliate 11Alive tells of VA's denial of benefits to many Camp Lejeune Veterans. (Faith Abubey 2019)

Deadly S.N.A.F.U.

See Chapter "Deny, Delay, Sickness and Death"

HIDDEN FACTS

On September 16, 2010 a Congressional hearing was held by members of the House of Representatives Committee on Science and Technology, Subcommittee on Investigations and Oversight. The hearing was titled, *Camp Lejeune: Contamination and Compensation, Looking Back, Moving Forward* and paints a bleak picture of the Marine Corps, the Department of the Navy, and others as being incompetent, knowingly hiding and obscuring evidence, not notifying hundreds of thousands that were impacted by the contaminated water, and in doing so inflicting great suffering and pain for many.

Beginning in October 1980 a series of tests were performed on the well water that was contaminated. Additional tests were made 1981 and 1982. All the tests indicated the water was contaminated with toxic chemicals. Marine officers in the chain of command were notified. Such stern warning comments in testers' reports as "water is highly contaminated with low molecular weight halo-generated hydrocarbons", etc. began appearing as early as 1980.

Deadly S.N.A.F.U.

In a reaction to test results provided by an outside testing laboratory, in 1982, the Base's Supervisory Chemist, who worked in the Quality Control Lab and had knowledge of the test results wrote "Trichloroethylene, like tetrachloroethylene and other halo-genated hydrocarbons (i.e., Trihalomethanes) at high levels, has been reported to produce liver and kidney damage and central nervous system disturbances in humans."

The answer to who knew what and when is now fairly well established. The Marine Corps knew in the early 1980's that the water was contaminated. I found no evidence that Navy doctors at the base hospital suspected contaminated water as being the cause of the many health issues that confronted them for over three decades. Finally, in 1984 and 1985 the wells were taken out of service due to contaminated volatile organic chemicals (VOCs) that are believed to have been in the water for over 30 years. The first announcement provided by the Marine Corps to base residents of contaminated water came in December 1984. Why did it take so long for the Marine Corps leadership to order the closure of the contaminated wells?

It wasn't until November 1988; the Department of the Navy issued a letter requesting ATSDR perform a health assessment at Camp Lejeune. Many years would pass when in 1991 ATSDR began a Public Health Assessment (PHA) and in October 1994 published its "Initial Release", and in 1997 its "Final Version". The final 1997 version stated:

``Volatile organic compound (VOC) levels in three base drinking water systems (Tarawa Terrace, Hadnot Point, and Holcombe Boulevard) were a health concern until 1985 when use of contaminated wells stopped. Well contamination was caused from leaks in off-base and on-base underground tanks that were installed in the 1940s and 1950s. Human exposure to trichloroethylene (TCE), tetrachloroethylene (PCE), and 1,2-dichloroethylene (DCE) in drinking water systems at MCB Camp Lejeune have been documented over a period of 34 months, but likely occurred for a longer period of time, perhaps as long as 30 years.''

The final 1997 PHA report had failed to address the issue benzene in Camp Lejeune's drinking water. There was one minor reference of benzene that appeared in a chart within the appendix of the report. However, in 1998 ATSDR did publish a report "Adverse Pregnancy Outcomes" that in part read ``Hadnot Point tap water,'' ``Nonetheless, low level exposure (an estimated 35 ppb) would have been expected among women receiving Hadnot Point water before December 1984.''

Deadly S.N.A.F.U.

Although the timeline of who knew what and when did they know it is still unfolding, we now have a fairly clear understanding. In 2009, the 1997 final PHA report was withdrawn from the ATSDR website when they acknowledged major flaws in that report. In 2009 new evidence was uncovered from the Department of the Navy regarding the large quantity of benzene that was leaked into the well water at Camp Lejeune.

As early as 1994 the ATSDR began writing to the Marine Corps that they were not receiving vital records regarding the full extent of the toxic contamination at Camp Lejeune. In 2005 the ATSDR informed the Government Accountability Office (GAO) there were a "substantial number of additional documents that had not been previously provided by Camp Lejeune officials."

In March 2009, the ATSDR stumbled across a previously undisclosed web portal belonging to the Navy. A sub-contractor to ATSDR was inadvertently given access to this portal by a Marine Corps' librarian. Contained within the NavFacEngCom's Underground Storage Tank (UST) web portal was documents previously withheld from the ATSDR including details on the size and scope of the fuel loss from the Hadnot Point Fuel Farm (HPFF) underground storage tanks. According to documents discovered in *the portal, the <u>Marine Corps lost 1.1 million gallons of</u>* *<u>fuel at the HPFF over the course of the 49-year</u>* *<u>operational history of the facility</u>. Much of this fuel was located within 300-1,100 feet away from well HP-602. The fuel was found at all levels in the aquifer including the deep aquifer. Where is the Navy's notification to ATSDR advising them of the existence of this portal and the 1.1 million gallons of fuel trapped in the ground at Hadnot Point?* What does the Navy and the Marine Corps stand to gain if the public, the scientists and Congress were not aware of the extreme nature of the loss fuel at the HPFF? (Hearing before Subcommittee on Investigations and Oversight, Serial #111-108 2010)

The documents uncovered by ATSDR in 2009 indicated between 1988 and 1991 there was 1.1 million gallons of gasoline floating on top of the groundwater table at Camp Lejeune. Water is heavier than gasoline. Fuel tanks at the base were leaking on average 21,200 gallons a year over many years. Benzene is a key component of gasoline and will eventually degrade into the water supply. The first documented fuel leak was in 1979 when an estimated 20,000 to 30,000 gallons of fuel leaked from an underground valve.

A condition survey for the HPFF was scheduled the following year and other problems were found at the

HPFF. The LantDiv engineer concluded that because of age, failure to clean the tanks, and lack of maintenance, there had been a general condition of corrosion and deterioration of the tanks and connecting pipelines. Many of the interconnecting valves and flanges could not be inspected because they were buried and/or could not be located. The engineer recommended replacing the connecting piping, the inspection of all of the tanks for leaks and repair existing leaks. The Condition Survey was followed in 1981 with a Military Construction Data project number LE201M to repair the HPFF facilities and $537,200 was then allocated to clean and repair the petroleum tanks. By March of 1983, Navy and Marine Corps officials determined that piecemeal rehabilitation of the HPFF was not cost effective and in 1985, the recommendation was made to replace the HPFF with a new facility. The fuel farm was finally replaced in 1990. (Hearing before Subcommittee on Investigations and Oversight, Serial #111-108 2010)

Serious fuel leaks were noted long before the wells were closed.

VICTIMS TESTIFY

MIKE PARTAIN

Mike Partain was diagnosed with male breast cancer at age 39 and was the first witness to testify at the House Subcommittee hearing on September 16, 2010. Mr. Partain was featured in the documentary *Semper Fidelis: Always Faithful* and has been a tireless advocate for those of us who drank and washed in the contaminated water or were impacted through birth. His parents lived at Camp Lejeune when his dad was an officer stationed there. He was conceived and born there. In his professional career he is an investigator for a major insurance company and has spent countless hours investigating the Camp Lejeune tragedy. Sometimes a few words can speak volumes. Mike Partain states, *"Trying to pin down the truth with the leadership of the Marine Corps is like trying to nail Jell-O to the wall."*

It is estimated by federal scientists that during the 30 plus years from August 1, 1953 through December 31, 1987 more than 2,500 babies may have been carried in utero on the base or born at Camp Lejeune Hospital. (B. Barrett, Warnings About Lejeune's Tainted Water Unheeded for Years 2010)

In the documentary Semper Fidelis: Always Faithful, Mike Partain and Jerry Ensminger are shown walking through a cemetery near the Base. There were numerous gravestones for very young babies and children. On several they assumed that at least one of the parents had been stationed at Camp Lejeune because a rank was carved into the gravestone when the name of the parents was shown.

COMMANDER JAMES L. WATTERS

The second witness to testify at the hearing was James L. Watters, a retired Naval officer, who served at the Naval Regional Medical Center at Camp Lejeune from June 1977 until November 1979. His service to his country is noteworthy. He served as an Army infantry man in Vietnam and was wounded in 1970. He then joined the Navy in 1975 was on active duty until 1981, and in the Naval Reserves from 1981 until 2000. He retired with the rank of Commander in the Naval Medical Service Corps.

His testimony was unsettling in that it reminded me of the same health issues that my best friend Jim Rogers had faced.

Commander Watters testifies, *"In November 2007, I was diagnosed with advanced renal cell carcinoma, stage 3, almost stage 4. I had a kidney removed in December 2007, and in January 2008 was told by my oncologist I had about a year to live. In approximately July 2008, I received an envelope from the IRS which contained a letter from General Payne advising me I had been exposed to trichlorethylene and other hazardous chemicals while serving at Camp*

Lejeune. It is important to note this letter came 21 years after the Marine Corps and the Department of the Navy knew in 1987 that I and many others had been exposed to volatile organic compounds."

Actually, his statement is incorrect, the Marine Corps knew of the problem in late 1980, also he seems unaware of the benzene issue that was uncovered a short time before his testimony. After being turned down twice for VA benefits, he received the important VA benefits on his third try.

Commander Watters continues in testimony, *"I would have appreciated being notified by the Marine Corps even 18 months before the July 2008 notice. It would have made a difference in when my kidney cancer was diagnosed and my prognosis. As I researched the Camp Lejeune situation, I was horrified to find out how many people the Marine Corps had poisoned and the obstructionist tactics the U.S. Marine Corps and Department of the Navy has used to avoid responsibility and avoid providing any type of assistance with health care or any financial assistance to those they have been sickened and to the families of those whose deaths they have caused. Examples of obstructionist tactics include the Marine Corps' failure to cooperate with the State of North Carolina's efforts to analyze and address this problem* *in the 1980s, the 21 years it took for the Marine Corps to notify those they poisoned, the intense pressure it took to have the Marine Corps fund the ATSDR study, the failure of the Marine Corps to turn over critical documents until forced to do so, and numerous other examples of the Marine Corps and Department of the Navy strategy to deny and delay as long as possible. I firmly believe this strategy is based upon financial considerations and I do not know what role the Department of Defense has in this strategy. It is possible that the Marine Corps and Department of the Navy senior leaders are `just following orders.' It is my firm belief that the United States Marine Corps and Department of the Navy leadership have abandoned and betrayed their wounded from Camp Lejeune including women and children and left them to suffer and die. I am very sensitive to caring for the wounded because in the Army we were trained to never leave our wounded behind. I saw men wounded and killed in Vietnam trying to recover our wounded. The U.S. Soldier's Creed specifically states, 'I will never leave a fallen comrade.' If the Marines have a similar creed, their senior leaders seem to think it does not apply in this case."*

Commander Watters had tried three times for VA benefits. He was successful the third time only after submitting letters from three medical experts from the school where he was assistant dean. He stated that his main objective was to obtain CHAMPVA insurance coverage for his family. (Hearing before Subcommittee on Investigations and Oversight, Serial #111-108 2010)

General Alfred M. Gray Jr. was the commanding officer of the 2nd Marine Division from June 5, 1981 until August 28, 1984, and Camp Lejeune is their home. There are about 19,000 Marines in a division. He later became Commandant of the Marine Corps (1987-1991). The failure to shut down the wells and lack of notification issues occurred under his watch either while Commanding General of the 2nd Division or as Commandant of the Marine Corps. Just some of his battlefield awards and commendations are worth noting: Silver Star, two awards Legion of Merit (V), four awards Bronze Star (V), three awards Purple Heart, etc. (Wikipedia n.d.)

My question would be when did the General, and then Commandant, first know of the problem and what did he do when he found out? Another question might be, how many in the chain of command that knew about the contaminated water drank it, washed in it, or let their families drink it and wash in it?

Deadly S.N.A.F.U.

PETER DEVEREUX

Another victim testifying was Peter Devereux. He was an enlisted man who served at Camp Lejeune from December 1980 until April 1982 and now had invasive ductal carcinoma, a very aggressive form of breast cancer. Like so many others who served at Camp Lejeune he had surgery and many chemotherapy and radiation treatments. The cancer has metastasized to his spine, ribs and hips. On August 1, 2008 he first received notification from the Department of the Navy of the Camp Lejeune water problem.

A timely notification would have prevented a tremendous amount of agony and sorrow and kept many from a premature and painful death. The pages of this book could contain hundreds, if not thousands, of horrific and similar stories. Nothing will be gained from sharing so many stories of pain and suffering.

Thank you to all who advocated on behalf of the thousands like myself who drank these poison cocktails. Whether a Marine or not, you are a thoughtful and passionate group of advocates. You have made a difference.

Mr. Devereux was asked if the Marines has a slogan similar to the Army's "Leave no comrade behind". His response *"Yes. You know, semper fidelis, always faithful, and you never leave a man behind, absolutely. Always protect your own."*

THE EXPERT

DR. RICHARD CLAPP

Dr. Clapp's background: Professor Emeritus, Department of Environmental Health, Boston University School (B.U.) of Public Health, Environmental Health Policy Consultant and Member of the ATSDR Camp Lejeune Community Assistant Panel (CAP) Dr. Clapp received his MPH degree from the Harvard School of Public Health in 1974 and his D.Sc. Degree in Epidemiology from B.U. School of Public Health in 1989.

Dr. Clapp states, *"The degree of contamination of drinking water at Camp Lejeune in the years between 1957 and 1985 is the highest I have observed in my career as an environmental epidemiologist. For example, the trichloroethylene concentration found in drinking water from one treatment plant in 1982 was 1,400 parts per billion. This is two hundred and eighty times the current allowable level of TCE in drinking water in the U.S. It is more than five times the highest level found in well water in Woburn, Massachusetts at about the same time as the childhood leukemia cluster was identified in that town."*

"... based on my experience as an epidemiologist, what types of health effects might be expected from this kind of contamination of these chemicals that have been documented and you documented, Mr. Chairman, and it would be in my view a variety of cancers, some of which have been mentioned here today--breast cancer in males and females, kidney cancer or renal cell carcinoma, non-Hodgkin's lymphoma, bladder cancer, and then some reproductive effects in the offspring including childhood cancer, in my view, and also adverse reproductive outcomes such as birth defects, small for gestational age children, et cetera,"

The Consultant

MICHAEL HARGETT

Mr. Hargett, was contracted by the Marine Corps to test the water at Camp Lejeune in 1982 and testified that he began notifying personnel at the base of contaminated water in that year. His notifications were made both in writing and through one-on-one meetings. At the time he was co-owner of Grainger Laboratories located in Raleigh, North Carolina. He holds a master's degree in Microbiology from North Carolina State University.

THE GOVERNMENT, ATSDR

CHRIS PORTIER

Director, Agency for Toxic Substances and Disease Registry Health Studies *Adverse Pregnancy Outcomes Reanalysis.*

In 1995, ATSDR began a study of adverse pregnancy outcomes at Camp Lejeune in relation to exposure to VOCs in drinking water. ATSDR found statistically significant associations for some subgroups (older mothers and mothers with histories of fetal loss) living in homes in Tarawa Terrace (PCE), and elevated risks of small for gestational age (SGA) births and low birth weights. Later information indicated that some women, who were considered not to be exposed because they were served by the Holcomb Boulevard system, were potentially exposed during pregnancy. ATSDR and the Department of Navy are engaged in intensive efforts to identify information needed for water modeling. ATSDR will conduct a new evaluation of adverse pregnancy outcomes when the modeled water concentrations are available. Case-Control Study of Specific Birth Defects and Childhood Cancers. ATSDR identified children born during 1968-1985 to mothers who were exposed to VOC-contaminated drinking water at Camp Lejeune at any time during their pregnancy. Cases of neural tube defects (i.e., spina bifida and anencephaly), cleft lip, cleft palate, leukemia or non-Hodgkin's lymphoma was identified during a telephone survey conducted during 1999-2002 and have been confirmed by medical records. The parents of confirmed cases and a random sample of controls (i.e., children who did not have birth defects or childhood cancers) were interviewed in 2005. Analyses of this data will be conducted once the results of the water modeling become available.

THE GENERAL

MAJOR GENERAL EUGENE G. PAYNE, JR.

Assistant Commandant, Excerpts from General Payne's written testimony before Senate Veterans' Affairs Committee on October 8, 2009. General Payne is a highly decorated Marine who first served at Camp Lejeune in 1970 as an enlisted man.

The underlined sentences were supplied by the author for emphasis.

HISTORY OF DISCOVERY

It is important to keep in mind that the events surrounding this situation occurred over 25 years ago. Environmental standards and regulations have changed dramatically over the intervening years as a result of advances in scientific knowledge and increased public awareness. The events at Camp Lejeune must be considered in light of the scientific knowledge, regulatory framework, and accepted industry practices that existed at the time, rather than in the context of today's standards. Trichloroethylene [TCE] and tetrachloroethylene [PCE] were discovered in the Camp Lejeune drinking water in the early 1980's. The circumstances that led up to the discovery are as follows. In 1981, Camp Lejeune officials became aware that VOCs were interfering with the analysis of potable water samples that were being collected in preparation for the implementation of future drinking water standards for Total Trihalomethanes (TTHM). Sampling conducted by a Navy contractor revealed that another chemical *present in the water sample was interfering with the analysis; however, the type of chemical and source were unknown. Base personnel continued to sample the water for TTHMs over the next several years using various laboratories with varying results. Through targeted sampling in 1982, two of Camp Lejeune's eight public drinking water systems were determined to be contaminated by two chemicals – TCE and PCE. TCE and PCE are chemicals commonly found in degreasing agents and dry-cleaning solvents respectively. It is important to note that there were no drinking water regulations in place for TCE, PCE, benzene, or vinyl chloride at the time of discovery. In the early 1980's, the Naval Assessment and Control of Installation Pollutants (NACIP) program, a precursor to the Department of the Navy (DON) Installation Restoration Program, was already in the process of identifying contaminated sites on Base for further sampling and investigation. Plans were in place to sample potable wells near the identified contaminated sites. It was these sampling events that identified, between late 1984 and early 1985, individual wells that contained groundwater impacted with TCE and PCE and other VOC's such as benzene. As the Base received sampling data on impacted wells, the wells were promptly removed from service. A separate investigation by the State of North Carolina in 1985 revealed leaks from an off-base dry cleaner had contaminated the wells near the Tarawa Terrace housing area. The Hadnot Point water system was contaminated by on-base sources. As referenced above, no drinking water standards for TCE or PCE were in place at the time of discovery, and all impacted wells were voluntarily removed from service promptly by Base direction in late 1984/early 1985. Initial regulation of these volatile organic compounds under the Safe Drinking Water Act did not begin until 1987. Final regulations on the chemicals were in force in 1989 and 1992 respectively.*

NOTIFICATION

Camp Lejeune first notified military personnel and family members about the impacted drinking water on December 13, 1984, through an article appearing in Camp Lejeune's newspaper, The Globe. Camp Lejeune also distributed a public notice to residents of Tarawa Terrace on April 30, 1985. In May 1985, Camp Lejeune issued a press release announcing the water contamination problem and explaining the steps being taken to restore water services to the affected base residents. Jacksonville Daily News and Wilmington Morning Star printed stories on the situation on May 11 and 12, 1985. In 2000, ATSDR requested assistance from the Marine Corps to reach additional participants for a survey they were conducting. At the time, the number of participants was approximately 6,500. ATSDR needed over 12,000 for a statistically valid study. The Marine Corps played an active role in assisting ATSDR in identifying participants eligible for the survey through both targeted and global notifications. In January 2000, Camp Lejeune held an "open house" with base residents and the Jacksonville community to discuss issues about the drinking water previously discovered to contain VOCs. In August 2000, Headquarters Marine Corps sent a message to all Marines worldwide in an effort to reach potential ATSDR survey participants. In addition, articles were published in numerous base newspapers including the Quantico Sentry, Camp Lejeune Globe, and Camp Pendleton Scout, which have a large readership of both active duty and retired military members. Camp Lejeune also solicited participants for the ATSDR survey by sending a press release to other military base publications. In November 2000, Headquarters Marine Corps held a press brief at the Pentagon asking media to assist in helping to reach survey participants. On January 25, 2001, Headquarters Marine Corps sent a second message to all Marines worldwide in an effort to reach potential ATSDR survey participants. In February 2001, regional media outreach efforts began, and outlets reached included: (A) TV Stations - 1027 outlets (B) Daily Newspapers - 1373 outlets (C) Weekly Newspapers - 1171 outlets

Total: 3571 media outlets contacted. In 2001, Headquarters Marine Corps requested approval from the Department of Defense to release to the ATSDR the Social Security numbers of potential survey participants. In July 2001, Headquarters Marine Corps received approval from DoD for a limited release of Social Security Number information covered by the Privacy Act to the ATSDR in order to support the ATSDR's survey participant location efforts. Based on extensive data searches by Headquarters Marine Corps, contact information for the names of potential survey participants was identified and forwarded to the ATSDR. The FY08 National Defense Authorization Act mandated that the Secretary of the Navy attempt to directly notify former residents of Camp Lejeune of their potential exposure to the chemicals. The Act also required that ATSDR develop a health survey to be included with the notification letter. On Sept. 14, 2007, the Marine Corps posted a link to the registration database on its website (www.marines.mil/clsurvey) so that former Camp Lejeune residents and workers as well as interested parties can be placed on a contact list to receive notification and information regarding this important issue. The call center became operational September 17, 2007 and is used as another tool to locate former residents and workers and register them to receive additional updates to the ongoing studies. In addition *to direct notifications, the Marine Corps continues to use various general communication venues to reach former base residents and workers to encourage them to register. This general notification has included articles and/or advertisements in newspapers such as USA Today, periodicals such as Time and Newsweek, internet advertisements on general consumer websites such as WebMD and Weather.com., military related websites such as the Leatherneck, U. S. Navy Institute, and the Vietnam Veterans Association, internet search engines such as Yahoo and Google, and radio broadcasts. <u>As of September 28, 2009, more than 140,000 individuals have been registered with the Marine Corps.</u>*

General Payne feels that the notification process was significant. I would argue that with only about 15% of those who served at Camp Lejeune registered as of September 28, 2009 the notification process had serious defects.

The Marine Corps has the social security numbers for all Marines who served at Camp Lejeune during the period from August 1, 1953 through December 31, 1987. The Internal Revenue Service, Medicare, and the Veterans Administration have powerful databases that can determine if someone is living or dead, their address, whether they are collecting VA benefits, etc. There is no excuse for the lack of timely notification to ALL the Marines and others who were poisoned at Camp Lejeune. The Marines began notifications on a very small scale in 1984. In 2008 Congress was well aware of the lack of notifications.

It was in early 2020, and not from the Marine Corps, that I first became aware of the seriousness of the problem and that in 2012 VA benefits now were available to qualified Reservists. Many who I served with died at early ages, some suffering horribly prior to death, many from diseases now presumed to have been caused from the contaminated water. It is my belief that many Marines have yet to be officially notified and in fact have no idea of this ongoing tragedy.

Included in General Payne's written testimony is his telling of how important the health and welfare of those poisoned are to the Marine Corps and why they are not at fault. His logic is the Marines are warfighters. What do they know about water contamination and notification?

He comments:

The health and welfare of our Marines, Sailors, their families, and civilian workers are a top priority *for the Marine Corps. The Marine Corps is and always has been a large family, and we all know people, including myself, who were stationed or worked at Marine Corps Base, Camp Lejeune during their military careers. The Marine Corps is deeply concerned with all the military and civilian families who are experiencing or have experienced any health issues and we understand that there are those who believe their health concerns may be a result of time spent at Camp Lejeune. The Marine Corps consists of war-fighters, and those who directly support warfighters. We have no epidemiological experts, and accordingly we rely on the expertise of scientific organizations like the Agency for Toxic Substances and Disease Registry (ATSDR) and the National Academies, National Research Council (NRC) to inform our understanding of this issue. We have provided over $14.5 million in funding and have exhausted countless man-hours in direct support of research initiatives. We will continue to support and cooperate with the Veterans Administration, the ATSDR and the NRC in an effort to get answers for those of our Marine Corps family who may have been exposed to volatile organic compounds (VOC) in drinking water at Camp Lejeune.*

General Payne had testified on September 9, 2009 before a House Sub-Committee on Investigations and Oversight. This is part of General

Payne's testimony during the question-and-answer period.

Mr. Broun. *Thank you, General. There have been many criticisms on how the Marine Corps, the Navy has responded to the contamination of the water supply there at Camp Lejeune. Looking back over the past 30 years is there any action or inaction that you would have changed?*

General Payne. *Sir, there are a number of actions that I would have changed. I would--I can't tell you how many times over the last three years in working with this issue on behalf of the Marine Corps, I would have given anything to have rolled back the clock and to have known and to have been able to influence during that era what we know today to be the case. It is astounding some of the things that happened, and I think that they happened for a number of reasons. I think part of it was mentioned earlier. I think we were ignorant, quite frankly, of some of the implications. I think we were lulled into a sense of complacency or at least a lack of urgency by the fact that we were not out of compliance. And I am not trying to excuse what happened. I think that there were many, many errors made on behalf of the Marine Corps. But it is difficult to look back through the lens of 2010 at what we did or did not know, or should or should not have done in the '60s, '70s, and early '80s, but there are many things that I would have done differently. There are things I would have done differently 5 and ten years ago. I have only been working this for about three years and it is--one normally shakes their head and wonders at some of the things that did or did not occur.*

(Hearing before Subcommittee on Investigations and Oversight, Serial #111-108 2010)

THE VETERANS ADMINISTRATION

THOMAS J. PAMPERIN

Associate Deputy Under Secretary for Policy and Program Management, Veterans Benefits Administration, U.S. Dept. of Veterans Affairs:

With specific respect to Camp Lejeune, VA does not operate a registry for this population or have special authority to enroll for health care veterans or their family members based upon service at Lejeune. The Marine Corps does have such a registry and VA has been working with DOD to get useful data for veterans who were stationed at Lejeune from the database. It has been estimated that approximately one million veterans and their dependents were assigned to Camp Lejeune during the period of the drinking water contamination. Veterans who are part of this cohort may apply for health care enrollment if *they are otherwise eligible and are encouraged to discuss any specific concerns with their health care provider. VA processes disability claims based on service at Camp Lejeune and possible exposure to chemical contaminants on a case by case basis. This approach has been adopted because the evidence to date on the long-term health effects due to potential contaminated drinking water at Lejeune is inconclusive. Establishing presumptive diseases at this point would be premature. <u>Approximately 200 claims have been received based upon service at Camp Lejeune and approximately 20 veterans thus far have been granted service-connection on a direct basis, most commonly for kidney diseases, non-Hodgkin's, and other cancers.</u> For those cases that have been denied, claims have normally not been granted because of one of three criteria: the veteran did not serve at Lejeune during the period of the contamination, the current disease, or disability and the medical nexus between the current disease was not established.* (Hearing before Subcommittee on Investigations and Oversight, Serial #111-108 2010)

This is a most telling statement of just how inept, ineffective and grossly negligent the Marine Corps was and is. They had the names of the about one million people who were at Camp Lejeune, they knew of the serious health problems that the contaminated water would cause and had caused, and for nearly thirty years the Marine Corps' actions to notify those poisoned were minimal at best. Finally, in 2008 Congress had to order notification to Marines. It is unimageable that in 2009, after so many years had passed, only approximately 200 claims had been filed with the VA and only approximately 20 received benefits.

Even after required to do so by a 2008 Federal law the notification process was largely inept and ineffective.

DENY, DELAY, SICKNESS AND DEATH

Anyone with a minimum knowledge of history would recognize the sacrifices that Marines have made in the service of this country. The Vietnam War was just one of many that the Marines fought in. It is mentioned here because the Marines involvement of 10 years took place from 1965 to 1975, that was within the time frame of the contaminated water issue at Camp Lejeune. I vividly remember that period. In 1965 I entered the Marine Corps, went to boot camp and then to Camp Lejeune. In 1965 the Marine Corps started to activate some of the more specialized reserve units but did not activate my reserve unit.

About 500,000 Marines served in Vietnam, nearly 15,000 were killed in action, and about 50,000 were wounded. Surely, many of these Marines had been stationed at Camp Lejeune during the period of contaminated water. The Marines have always paid the price, but has our government?

In 2008 a federal law was enacted that required the Department of the Navy to notify Marines who had been stationed at Camp Lejeune during the between 1958-1987 of the dangers of the contaminated water. In 2009 the VA indicated that only 200 Marines had filed claims for benefits, and only 20 had received benefits. In 2012 a law was enacted that provided VA health care benefits for Marines who had certain presumptive diseases, and in 2017 VA disability benefits were added. However, the number of presumptive diseases were reduced for disability claim.

Between January 2011 and June 2019, 84,000 Camp Lejeune water contamination claims were filed with the VA. Although the VA indicated to 11Alive (Atlanta's NBC affiliate) that 74% were approved on presumptive conditions, 11Alive requested and received data from the VA. From the data received 11Alive determined that less than 25% of the claims were approved.

The VA placed a roadblock into the Lejeune veteran claim process by requiring all claims to be evaluated by a "Subject Matter Expert" (SME). Little is known as how the SME's are chosen or how they operate. However, the grant rate dropped from 25% to 8%. It seemed obvious to even a casual observer that the SME simply provided another way to delay and deny benefits. On December 7, 2015 three veterans' groups under the Freedom of Information Act (FOIA) requested information from the VA and when no information was received, they filed a lawsuit in Federal court. On February 27, 2018 Judge

Victor A. Bolden of the U.S. District Court of Connecticut ordered the VA to show cause why it should not be held in contempt. Veterans, like myself thank the Yale Law School's Veterans Legal Services Clinic for their efforts on our behalf. (School 2018)

"It sounds to me like it's the kind of process that is often used by insurance companies where you really have to fight for your benefits, even though the right for those benefits is pretty obvious to everybody else around," Dr. Shay said. "It's amazing how the system works. People just deny and deny and deny that harm was done to somebody."

"I think it's obviously a system that is not working to the benefit of the people who have been in the military and protected us all," Dr. Shay explained. "We live in a world where we don't acknowledge the responsibility of the government to take care of things that they caused, and or to support those people who have been at the front lines."

Dr. Robert Shay had been Willie Copeland's doctor for 15 years. Mr. Copeland had been stationed at Camp Lejeune for two and a half years in the 1980's and now suffered from kidney disease. He had lost both his legs from the disease and now had only one functioning kidney. Apparently, the VA wanted conclusive proof of kidney cancer and Dr. Shay, fearful that a biopsy could damage his one good kidney did not perform one. The VA had rejected Copeland's application for benefits three times over a six-year period.

"The VA has never contacted me, personally, to ask me for my records or to ask me about what I perceive to be his issues. So, they are missing a major link. I mean, I've been his nephrologist since 2004," the doctor explained. (Faith Abubey 2019)

By the time the Public Law was enacted in 2008 Public Law that required the Navy to notify or <u>make a best effort to</u> notify those veterans impacted many years (over twenty), had now passed, and many had died as a result of the poisons contained in the water. Now, an investigative article by 11Alive further illustrates just how poorly the Marine Corps performed the notification process. In 2009, the VA testified that only about 200 Camp Lejeune water contamination claims had been received. Since the 2008 Public Law required notification the number of claims grew dramatically. In a nine-year period after notifications were required 84,000 VA claims were filed.

It also gives more clarity to just how serious and deadly the situation is and how important early notification would have been. Typically, the sooner someone becomes aware of a potential medical problem, the sooner they can react to mitigate the risk and reduce the negative health issues. Now, after many years have passed, 84,000 very sick Marines or their dependents had filed claims for VA benefits. It would be fair to assume that many of these 84,000 had become sick long prior to the 2008 Public Law requiring either direct notification or a best effort. It is also fair to assume that many had died prior to notification and no VA claims were made.

It is my best guesstimate that more than 100,000 members of the Marine Corps Active Reserves had served at least 30 days at Camp Lejeune during the identified time frame of over 30 years. The calculation is fairly straight forward. My best estimate is that at least 10% of the about 1,000,000 who were living or stationed at Camp Lejeune were Active Reserves.

There are about 40,000 Marine Active Reserves that are stationed at 184 Reserve Training Centers located throughout the United States. There about 185,000 Marines on active duty. (Wikipedia n.d.)

<u>It is also my belief that the Active Reserves have never been directly notified by the Navy, Marine Corps, or any government agency of Lejeune's water issues</u>.

If Dr. Shay's comments are to be believed, and I feel strongly they are correct, the government's position is to delay and deny. As brave Marines, their families and others suffer and die, the Department of the Navy, the Marine Corps, and the Veterans Administration must know that as time passes the bulk of the problems will eventually go away. If about one million people were exposed to this poisoned water, and so many years have now passed, and the VA has only paid healthcare or disability benefits to about 20,000 people as of 2019, the government will have paid very little to help resolve a catastrophic problem that they created. Certainly, good health would have been preferred, but that was and is not possible for so many who drank and washed in that poison.

Besides VA benefits, many victims or their estates were suing the Navy in civil court for damages. Then in 2019 the Navy denied all remaining civil claims. The following article by NBC news explains the Navy's justification for denying these civil claims.

The secretary of the Navy is denying all remaining civil claims by individuals **exposed to contaminated drinking water at Camp Lejeune in North Carolina**, *leaving roughly 4,500 plaintiffs with claims of more than $963 billion in damages with no cash payouts.*

In an exclusive interview with NBC News, Secretary of the Navy Richard Spencer defended the decision, saying the law does not support the claims.

"There is no legal way for the Department of the Navy to pay damages in these cases," Spencer said. _"We are denying the claims to free everybody to take their own course of action."_

Spencer acknowledged this will be "tremendously difficult" for the veterans and their families, who will have little chance of receiving a large monetary payout for their losses. Individuals have six months to appeal the decision.

The first argument for denying civil claims is based on a North Carolina law that sets a strict timeline of 10 years for an injured party to file a civil claim. The law applies even if the injured party is not aware of the exposure until after the 10-year deadline. Because the wells at Camp Lejeune were closed in 1985, the deadline for filing passed in the late 1990s.

The second argument for dismissing all the Camp Lejeune claims is based on an exemption to the Federal Tort Claims Act called discretionary function, which protects the U.S. government from lawsuits in cases in which negligence was not clearly established. In the case of Camp Lejeune, no one was instructed to cut off the water supply, so there's no clear case of negligence, according to Spencer.

The final argument is based on the Feres doctrine, a policy that prevents military members from suing *the federal government for injuries incurred during their service.*

Spencer said he was briefed on the legal limitations to the claims as soon as he took office 17 months ago. "It became apparent we had to make a decision," he said. Otherwise, he added, the claimants are being kept "in limbo."

During a news conference Thursday announcing the decision, Spencer said he couldn't answer why any of his predecessors didn't make the decision. "I wanted to come to closure on this," he said. "Kicking it down the road provided no value."

Spencer added that claimants can "work with Congress" to see if they can add benefits besides health care and disability. (Courtney Kube 2019)

As a side note, I remember a conversation I had with a friend and fellow reservist years ago at the training center. He was a truck driver and had struck and killed a pedestrian. His attorney told him that as far as monetary damages it was often far less costly to kill someone than to seriously injure them. I think of that comment often as I write this book.

TOXIC VAPOR INTRUSIONS DIDN'T END IN 1987!

Camp Lejeune is a massive Marine Corps base having over 14,000 structures on about 246 square miles. Thousands of Marines and others have either lived or worked in one building or another daily. The drinking and washing in the contaminated water may have ended in 1987, but the dangers from breathing poisonous vapors that had seeped into any one of the thousands of buildings continued. Vapor intrusion (VI) as it is called, are vapors released into buildings from the toxic volatile chemicals that have saturated the soil or are released from contaminated the ground water. The illusion that Lejeune was safe after 1987 was just that, an illusion. After the wells were finally closed for good in 1987 Camp Lejeune remained an active military base.

Toxic volatile organic chemicals (VOC) are a class of chemicals that start to evaporate at low temperatures and release poisonous vapors. The chemicals, are lighter than water, sit on top of the water and their vapors travel upward through the soil. Over time the plumes of poisonous vapors increase in size, spread over more land mass, and intrude into more structures.

Breathing toxic vapors is as dangerous to your health as drinking or washing in the contaminated water. Eye irritation, respiratory irritation, headaches and nausea are just some of the symptoms that can occur. Depending on the chemicals in the building and the length of exposure, the risk of cancer or chronic disease can increase dramatically. The Connecticut Department of Health released a technical health brief that listed VOC's of greatest concern for vapor intrusion. Some of the chemicals found in fuel released into the soil and water from a fuel tank leak are benzene, toluene, ethylbenzene, xylene and MTBE and can lead to a higher health risk of leukemia, nervous system disorders, reproductive disorders, kidney damage, and other diseases. TCE and PCE can lead to a higher risk of cancer, birth defects, kidney toxicity, and nervous system disorder. Vinyl chloride leads to a higher risk of cancer. All the above toxic chemicals and more are found in the soil and water at Camp Lejeune. (Health 2012)

The use of taking a canary into a coal mine to alert miners of the existence of carbon monoxide and other toxic gases began in 1911 and ended in 1986 when a detector with a digital reading replaced the canaries. If the miners noticed that the canary had become sick or had died the miners knew that an odorless toxic gas had intruded into their mine. It was time for miners to immediately leave the dangerous area that they were in. The known dangers of toxic vapor intrusions have been well known long before Camp Lejeune came into existence in 1943. (Eschner 2016)

Reports of smelling toxic vapors in buildings at Camp Lejeune continued long after the wells were finally closed in 1987. With that said, some toxic vapors, i.e., TCE, are odorless.

A chronology compiled by advocates Jerry Ensminger, Jim Fontella, and Mike Pertain contain a listing of about 50 documents and scientific reports generated relating to toxic vapor intrusions into many buildings at Camp Lejeune and the imminent dangers from toxic plumes near or under existing buildings. The chronology lists documents and reports issued over two decades, from May 1, 1988 through August 15, 2010. In their introduction to the chronology the authors indicated the documents and reports had been obtained from the State of North Carolina. The USMC/Navy leadership either had received or issued most, if not all, of the listed documents and was aware of the dangers of toxic vapor intrusions. (Jerry Ensminger n.d.)

Just several of the many documents listed:

August 1, 1988, Colonel Dalzell, U. S. Marine Corps Assistant Chief of Staff Marine Corps Base

Camp Lejeune requested the Hospital's Preventive Medicine to address air monitoring in selected buildings for VOC's within the Hadnot Point Industrial area. On August 25, 1988 Naval Hospital responded it did not have staff and was unable to perform requested testing.

April 30, 1998, a report prepared by Catlin Engineering for the Navy indicated buildings 1100, 1103, 1108, and 1115 were at risk from petroleum hydrocarbon vapors. Because of underground plumes beneath it, building 1005 had been evacuated several times due to the presence of petroleum hydrocarbon vapors.

June 28, 2002 the air sparging system in building 1101 had been shut down since November 2001. Vapors were detected in the building October 2001.

Reporter William R. Levesque's article on Lejeune and vapor intrusion monitoring found no evidence of vapor testing at the base before the late 1990's. The Navy indicated that records may have been destroyed, which would have been in violation of regulations. (W. R. Levesque 2011)

The following appeared in a detailed report prepared and published in March 2016 for the USMC and Navy leadership by a well-recognized engineering consulting firm:

MCB Camp Lejeune initiated a Basewide vapor intrusion (VI) evaluation in 2007 to identify buildings where VI might be occurring and to evaluate potential risks posed to building occupants from VI related to groundwater impacts. The phased VI evaluation indicated that, although VI was not a significant pathway of concern at the buildings investigated, there was a potential for the VI pathway to become significant at Site 88 (Buildings 3, 3B, 37, and 43), Site 78 (Building 902), and the Hadnot Point Fuel Farm (HPFF) (Buildings 1005 and 1115) in the future. Based on the results of the evaluation, MCB Camp Lejeune elected to install a VIMS in each of the seven buildings in February 2012. Performance monitoring began in March 2012 and has been conducted quarterly since then. (Vapor Intrusion Mitigation System(VIMS) Performance Monitoring... n.d.)

Tens of thousands of Marines and others had worked or passed through dozens of buildings where the likelihood of toxic vapor intrusions existed. There were numerous complaints of fuel fumes in buildings both before and after the last well was closed in 1987, with some buildings having to be evacuated. Again, it should be noted that some vapors were odorless.

The Agency for Toxic Substances and Disease Registry (ATSDR) had created a community assistance panel (CAP) for the Camp Lejeune site. The purpose of the CAP is to voice the concerns of the affected community of Marines and their families and to provide input on ATSDR's public health activities. Members of the CAP provided individual input as well as representing the views of the community and groups to which they belong. ATSDR considered the views expressed by CAP members during the ATSDR decision making process. The first meeting was held in February 2006 with meetings continuing since then. Vapor intrusion was discussed many times. (Camp Lejeune Community Assistance Panel (CAP) Meeting January 15, 2015)

The following is an exchange between ATSDR environmental epidemiologist Dr. Angela Ragin and CAP member Christopher Orris at the CAP meeting held on January 15, 2015:

DR. RAGIN: [*This is*] *the next action item assigned to the Department of the Navy. The CAP wants to know, in light of the July 9, 2014, EPA Region 9 memorandum, is the Navy/Marine Corps planning to personally notify women at Camp Lejeune who may have been in the past or might now currently be exposed to TCE via vapor intrusion. The CAP recommends this notification include all buildings over the TCE plume, and especially the 12 buildings currently being investigated for vapor intrusion. Immediate communication should occur with current workers and residents who are potentially exposed*

119

now to explain the recent EPA memorandum recommendations. I will read the response from the Department of the Navy. Their response: Following the EPA guidelines, comprehensive vapor intrusion studies are going on at several locations on Camp Lejeune for multiple groundwater contaminants including TCE. The EPA Region 9 memorandum provides additional information on TCE, and relevant portions have been incorporated to a complex decision-making process for vapor intrusion studies on Camp Lejeune. If a comprehensive assessment suggests potential vapor intrusion concerns for TCE or other compounds on Camp Lejeune, the Marine Corps will provide fact sheets and plan for appropriate follow-up on managers to the building occupants in a timely manner.

MR. ORRIS: *So, it's my understanding that exposure to TCE -- for a woman who is of child-bearing age exposure can cause a cardiac defect in as little as one day with exposure. And we are looking at possible buildings for vapor intrusion. I think now this response is very lacking.*

The number of hazardous sites at the massive military base almost defies imagination. In 2017 it was reported that there were 227 hazardous sites with final cleanup completion expected in 2057, covering hundreds of acres and spread throughout the base. Some sites are protected only by fencing with no remediation taking place, while others have ongoing remediation activities. As time passes the size of some toxic plumes has grown. The dangers have increased. (Camp Lejeune MCB December 5, 2017)

ABC Cleaners dumped hazardous solvents such as PCE, also known as PERC, through a leaky septic system for nearly 50 years. ABC was placed on the EPA's Superfund list in 1989. Water that supplied two of Lejeune's wells at Tarawa Terrace which in part supplied about 6,200 residents at a base housing community was contaminated from ABC's solvents. Because of budget cuts, bankruptcies and legal disputes, cleanup efforts in 2020 were at a standstill. Over time the size of the toxic plume has increased. The site will continue to be a major source of contamination for years to come. (Sorg 2020)

In 2020 the ATSDR announced they will perform a vapor intrusion health assessment for Camp Lejeune. Because of limitations, the ATSDR will evaluate about 190 buildings out of about 14,000 structures. About 33 of those buildings will be residences, of which about 11 are considered child activity buildings. They expect the assessments to be completed in 2022. It will then have been 35 years since the last well was closed in 1987. (ATSDR 2020)

Ask yourself, why would the ATSDR wait so long to do such a costly and time-consuming health assessment and what would you expect the results to be? Just based on my research, I believe that as new information was developed and old documents came to light, the ATSDR became gravely concerned.

Marines and others that were at Lejeune after 1987 now have or will face serious health issues. They were never notified that they would be working or living in buildings that jeopardized their good health. In fact, most still are not aware of the dangers they faced. Sadly, many will become sick and die not knowing that it is more likely than not that they were poisoned from toxic vapors.

This 2021 Facebook reply came from a woman Marine to a post on a Camp Lejeune group page. The question that was posed, did the poisoning finally stop in 1987?

Her reply was *"That's what I'm saying!!! I was there in 1995 and have a liver disease that they can't explain how I got."*

THE MARINES' HYMN

From the Halls of Montezuma
To the shores of Tripoli;
We fight our country's battles
In the air, on land, and sea;
First to fight for right and freedom
And to keep our honor clean;
We are proud to claim the title
Of United States Marine.

Our flag's unfurled to every breeze
From dawn to setting sun;
We have fought in ev'ry clime and place
Where we could take a gun;
In the snow of far-off Northern lands
And in sunny tropic scenes;
You will find us always on the job
The United States Marines.

Here's health to you and to our Corps
Which we are proud to serve;
In many a strife we've fought for life
And never lost our nerve;
If the Army and the Navy
Ever look on Heaven's scenes;
They will find the streets are guarded
By United States Marines.

The Marines' Hymn still gives me a chill every time I hear it sung; the music alone inspires me. It tells a story of how the Marines have fought all over the world, for what is right, for freedom, and to keep their honor clean. It goes on to wish you and the Corps good health.

Think about it, the good health of so many has been destroyed. Many have died. Many more will eventually become horribly sick and die from drinking and washing in the contaminated water. Some of their children, who have never set foot on the base, will face many of the same terrible health problems.

How incredibly sad!

JOINT BASE PEARL HARBOR-HICKAM
ANOTHER WATER CONTAMINATION TRAGEDY

Beginning in 1984, as part of the environmental cleanup program, some drinking water wells were tested near potential former disposal sites. <u>Benzene, a volatile organic compound (VOC), was found in one of the wells serving the Hadnot Point water system. When Base officials were notified of the result, the well was taken out of service on the same day it was found to be affected, and a more comprehensive well testing effort began.</u>

The above paragraph was copied directly from a pamphlet titled "Camp Lejeune Historic Drinking Water" published by the Department of the Navy, United States Marine Corps. I received the pamphlet directly from the Marine Corps in April 2020.The Marine Corps has been part of the Department of the Navy since 1834. Although, I had printed this paragraph in the first chapter of this book, it is important that it be reprinted here.

In the relatively short text above we are told several important facts. There was **testing of drinking water** at Camp Lejeune **in 1984**, **benzene** (a chemical **found in many petroleum-**

based fuels) was discovered in one well, and that well was **taken out of service the same day.**

However, the paragraph is misleading in one respect. The benzene that contaminated the water entered the aquifer from fuel that had leaked, over a period of years, from archaic and poorly maintained leaky underground fuel storage tanks located near the well in question. It was not a disposal site.

As the Red Hill disaster begins being told, ask yourself who knew what, when did they know it, and what did they do about it when they found out.

It is now May 2022, almost two years after this book was first published. In late December 2021, through a newspaper article, I first became aware of fuel leaks from a massive underground fuel tank storage area known as Red Hill at Joint Base Pearl Harbor-Hickam (JBPHH) in Oahu, Hawaii. (Alex Horton 2021) Although the magnitude of this disaster is still unknown, I have every reason to believe JBPHH will be as bad, if not worse, than the Camp Lejeune contaminated water tragedy.

Joint Base Pearl Harbor-Hickam (JBPHH) is a huge military base that is located eight miles from Honolulu on the Hawaiian Island of Oahu. A base merger in 2010 combined Naval Station Pearl Harbor and Hickam Air Force Base and the joint base now houses branches of the Navy, Air Force, Army and Coast Guard. Many of those serving at the base have their families living in base housing. The massive base is located on about 30,000 acres, with over 4,200 facilities, four dry docks, 31 piers, and a population of about 93,000 military and their families. (Guide 2018)

All of the JBPHH potable water, and until recently about 77% of the potable water for the Island of Oahu came from the Oahu Sole Source Aquifer. A Sole Source Aquifer is an aquifer that has been designated by the United States Environmental Protection Agency as the sole or principal source of drinking water for an area. By definition, Sole Source Aquifer is an aquifer that supplies at least 50% of the drinking water consumed in the area overlying the aquifer. The water had been designated as safe drinking water under the Federal Safe Drinking Water Act and those drinking, washing and swimming in it have every expectation that it would be safe. It is highly probable that water pumped from the Oahu Sole Source Aquifer has not been safe to drink or wash in for decades. (DeNovio 2021)

Not far from JBPHH main side and a part of the base is the Red Hill Mountain Range underground fuel storage facility. Unlike any other facility in the United States, Red Hill can store up to 250 million gallons of fuel. When first built, it consisted of 20 quarter inch steel-lined underground storage tanks (UST), encased in concrete, and built into cavities that were mined inside of Red Hill Mountain. The 20 tanks at Red Hill measure 100 feet in diameter and are 250 feet in height. Each tank has a storage capacity of approximately 12.5 million gallons. This is the largest underground fuel storage area in the United States.

The Red Hill tanks are connected to three gravity-fed pipelines that run 2.5 miles inside a tunnel to fueling piers at Pearl Harbor. (Jedra, How The Red Hill...Threatened Oahu's Drinking water 2021)

On November 20, 2021 about 14,000 gallons of jet fuel had spilled inside an access tunnel providing fire suppression and service lines for the Red Hill fuel storage facility. It was likely the result of operator error. Almost immediately residents on base started becoming horribly sick. They had been drinking and washing in water contaminated with jet fuel. Breathing its toxic vapors was also sickening. Pets were dying. Some pets, early on, simply stopped drinking the water. Social media and the newspapers began telling in real time what the families were going through. About 9,000 households were affected and about 3,500 military families were temporarily moved off base. (Jowers, CDC wants to hear... 2022) (BenZvi 2022)

Soon Facebook posts and newspaper articles began appearing. JBPHH residents began telling in real time of their own personal dire situation. Several comments follow:

Daisy Mortensen Stickney (Zay is her daughter) wrote,

As I ponder where to start with an update, my mind is overloaded. Since I decided to go public on the 21st, We have not stopped fighting. Everyday. And some nights. Phone calls, constant doc appointments, lots of writing and researching and talking to any news reporter who reaches out. We've had a total of 22 appointments, more than half just for Zay. Two trips by ambulance to the ER. Of course, the normal things too. You know, eating, hygiene, being a parent.

Zay is about the same. Still fainting, still seizing. Her life has consisted of sleeping, doctor appointments, testing, labs, time on the floor, and sleeping. More appointments, testing and labs coming up this next week. She now has to use a walker, which is just so heartbreaking to watch.

Jamie Simic wrote this shortly after leaving Hawaii. She started becoming ill while at JBPHH and prior to the November 20, 2021 acknowledged leak.

I am being discharged after 7 days in the hospital. Yes, I was diagnosed with hydrocarbon and carcinogen toxicity. I had surgery on esophagus while here along with countless MRI's, blood draws and urinalysis. I will have to repeat my esophageal procedure every 2 months. Unfortunately, it is not a permanent fix. I have 2 more surgeries minimum that need to be done ASAP but my children need me. I am 2 hours away from them right now, one way...Smelling fresh air as well as touching clean water is something that I cannot begin to describe. I have a very long road ahead of me.

Shari Shaaf Lichau also became sick prior to the November 20, 2021 leak. Her son also became very sick.

I am sick again, this time it's even more violent than before. I have nausea, am throwing up, sweating, can't handle caught a breath, shaking uncontrollably and I am heading to the Dr. Again @ DoD Navy, they still refuse to test me properly, my husband has had enough. He wants a diagnosis, as does everyone else on the Island. I just wanted to keep you informed. I will probably have to leave the Island without my husband all thanks to the DoD, Navy and DoH (Department of Health) who feel that black water is all clear. They still haven't shut tunnels down fully, still using them. The people of Hawaii are breaking down. It's just awful and heartbreaking to see families being tore apart.

In the first three months of 2022 almost every post in the JBPHH Facebook group was from someone who was horribly sick. More often than not other members of their family, especially children were also very sick. When such a post appeared responses would follow with others telling of their own difficult health situation.

As at Camp Lejeune high ranking military officers downplayed the enormity of the tragedy that was unfolding.

Residents started reporting oil products in the water on or about November 28, 2021. It wasn't until December 3, 2021 that the Navy confirmed there was a problem. Soon after, the public was made aware that on November 20, 2021, 14,000 gallons of jet fuel had spilled into the water.

Navy Captain Erik Spitzer, base commander made the following public statement in an email to base residents on November 29, 2021, "My staff and I are drinking the water on the base this morning, and many of my team live in housing and drink and use the water as well. There are no immediate indications that the water is not safe." A week later on December 5th he wrote an apology for making the statement and acknowledged the water was not safe. (Jowers, "I regret I did not tell..." 2021)

One Facebook reaction to Spitzer's apology came from Jen Johnston, *"While the written apology is appreciated, the blatant gaslighting of residents and dependents caused direct, verifiable, physical harm. Residents TRUSTED you and continued to consume contaminated water,"*

Army Major Amanda Feindt told Congressional members in February 2022, *"I'm here as a mother of two children who were poisoned on American soil by an American asset. I believe the Navy failed our children; I believe it was negligent."* Both Major Feindt and her 4-year-old daughter wound up in the hospital. She had been reassured that the water was safe and a week later found out it was not.

Navy Captain Michael McGinnis, Pacific Fleet Surgeon told Congressional lawmakers in January 2022 that medical providers had screened 5,900 patients with symptoms such as nausea and vomiting, headaches, diarrhea, skin and eye irritation, that are consistent with acute environmental exposure. He went on to say once the patients were removed from the water the symptoms *"rapidly resolved"*. (Jowers, Navy cites "operator error'... 2022)

Any family that has lived through the Camp Lejeune tragedy would be taken back by Captain McGinnis's comments. Those of us who drank and washed in the toxic water are at a significantly higher risk of facing serious long term health issues. Many are now very sick, and many have died from diseases presumed to have been caused by the contaminated water.

In early 2022 residents living in certain areas on the base were given the all clear by the Navy to return to their homes. The Navy indicated the water was now good to drink and wash in. Facebook post videos soon started to appear showing what seemed to be oil slicks on top of the water. Veronica Crescioni posted on May 5th *"I have hesitated to share my experience last week because I was so shook. But here we go...I took a bath, shower and brushed my teeth Sunday the 24th with our homes own water. Up until this point I've been taking camp showers with bottled water since we were sent home from our hotel mid-March. We've had our home flushed multiple times in the past couple months and were told by the Navy we were good to go after having a full panel water test done on our home. I didn't want to test it on the kids so I was the guinea pig. Headache, itchy skin and scalp, burning lips and throat and nausea all by Monday morning! One bath, one shower...but it didn't stop there. My symptoms improved after a clean water camp shower on Monday and laying low the next couple days. By Thursday all that was left is a throat that felt like I was swallowing an egg every time I swallowed my own spit. My PCM on base told me to go to the Urgent Care and from Urgent Care they sent me to the ER. Swabbed negative for everything...CT showed no lumps on my epiglottis. Given lots of meds to take care of the inflamed epiglottis so I could breathe easier. I was told that they were putting down my experience with the water as possible cause. It has been a rough week carrying on and healing.*

DO NOT USE THE WATER. CALL AND COMPLAIN!"

In May 2022, the Hawaii Department of Health released new maps showing the underground movement of the petroleum plume. The maps reflected both an increase in size of petroleum plume and what appears to be westward movement. Marti Townsend, former director of the Sierra Club of Hawaii commented, "I was shocked, speechless just to see the extent of contamination and how severe it was is really quite startling." (Richardson, State show "disturbing" ...plume maps 2022)

A March 31, 2016 article titled "Crude Oil Byproducts in Groundwater Plumes" published by the United States Geological Survey states that petroleum hydrocarbon fuel spills produce byproducts known as metabolites that are more soluble in the groundwater than the original crude oil. These metabolites, or oil breakdown byproducts, also are toxic and can cause serious negative health consequences. The plume of water-soluble metabolites expands more rapidly than the non-degraded petroleum hydrocarbon fuel plume that is lighter than the water it floats on it. Water moves differently and at different speeds than a petroleum hydrocarbon fuel plume.

Rear Admiral Blake Converse, Deputy Commander of the Pacific Fleet stated in his testimony at a House Armed Services subcommittee in January 2022, "The Navy caused the problem. We own it, and we're going to fix it." (Gonzalez 2022)

Admiral Blake Converse's comments are somewhat correct, the Navy did cause the problem, but the damage caused to the environment and to the health of so many is simply not fixable now nor will it ever be fixable.

Unfortunately, the problem covers many decades of petroleum leaks, spills, neglect, mismanagement, lies, secrecy, and misinformation.

An analysis issued by the Navy in 2009 indicated that if only 16,000 gallons of fuel leaked from the Red Hill fuel farm it could poison the Oahu aquifer with benzene, a known carcinogen.

A Navy consultant in 2018, in a report, stated that there is a 27.6 percent chance that in any given year 30,000 gallons could leak, and there was a chronic risk of over 5,800 gallons of fuel leaking each year. (Jedra, How The Red Hill...Threatened Oahu's Drinking water 2021)

Like at Camp Lejeune, the Navy was neither open nor transparent about what was taking place at the Red Hill fuel farm. Although the Navy knew of fuel releases for decades, the public did not. The facility had been considered classified and independent investigations did not begin to take place until 1995. What independent investigators discovered by piecing together historical Navy documents was that during a period of about 40 years, the early 1940's until early 1980's, about 180,000 gallons of fuel had leaked or been spilled.

At about same the time the wells at Camp Lejeune were shut down in the 1980's the Navy stopped documenting the Red Hill facility leaks or spillages. The non-documentation of leaks, with one exception in 1998, lasted until 2014. In 2014 a large spill of 27,000 gallons was recorded, so for a period of over 30 years, early 1980 to about 2014, Navy records show practically no leakage or spillage. This is not believable. (DeNovio 2021)

Since first built in 1940's and until the early 1980's there had been about 70 Red Hill documented leaks or spills. Yet, in February 2021 Navy Commander Darrel Frame testified under oath that except for the 2014 event there had been no fuel releases since 1988. (Jedra, Amid 'politcal concerns' Navy kept quiet... 2021)

In October 2021 a Navy officer, an unnamed whistleblower, told the Hawaii Department of Health that Navy officials gave false testimony and withheld information about corrosion at the Red Hill facility. The officer reported historical records of corrosion and leaks are being hidden from regulators. (Jedra, Whistleblower says Navy gave false testimony... 2021)

t.

Also, in 2021 Hawaii fined the Navy $325,000 for maintenance and operation violations. Inspection of the fuel tanks by the Navy were often unreliable and at times just didn't take place. Eight of the twenty tanks had not been inspected in over 20 years.

Navy Captain Albert Hornyak was fired in 2022 from his position as commanding officer of Naval Supply Systems Command Fleet Logistics Center after he warned his commanding officer of pressure surges and stated "I believe there are multiple valves in the Red Hill pipeline system are potentially leaking." His email comment was made public. (Richardson, Fired Navy captain privately raised concerns... 2022)

In March 2022 the Department of Defense announced that the Red Hill fuel tank storage facility will be permanently shut down. The Navy was required by the Hawaii Health Department, as part of an emergency order, to have an independent assessment of the facility. The firm Simpson Gumpertz and Heger Inc. (SGH) conducted the assessment and in late April 2022 published their 880-page assessment report. SGH indicated that the facility was in such a poor state and it may take up to two years just to safely start defueling. Some of the issues that were found; heavily corroded structural columns and pipes, concrete cracking and spalling, leakage through the tunnel walls and floor, valves known to leak, and the need for lead abatement in many areas. The problems exist from the fuel storage area at Red Hill to the final distribution point some 2.5 miles away at Pearl Harbor.

Like at Camp Lejeune, just based on the records available, and the time frames involved, estimated chronic annual leakage, corrosion and degradation at the Red Hill facility, an estimate can be made of the total amount of fuel leaked or spilled. My estimate would be that over 450,000 gallons of fuel has leaked or spilled into the aquifer since the facility was first built in the early 1940's.

This would include the 48,000 gallons of fuel that spilled during a 1948 earthquake, the accumulated documented leakage amount of 180,000 gallons from 1940's until the early 1980's, and a chronic annual leakage estimate of about of about 5,800 gallons a year for 42 years starting in 1980 through 2021.

Also, and most disturbing, the Department of Navy states that the well at Camp Lejeune was closed the same day that benzene, through chemical analysis, was found in the water. That was in the mid-1980's, but the chemical sampling of the Oahu (Red Hill) aquifer water didn't begin until about 1998, well over a decade later. (Jedra, Consultant: Fixing Red Hill's Decrepit Infrastructure... 2022)

There is evidence that when a large spillage occurs that water taken from the well nearest the fuel farm had significantly spiked with levels of toxic chemicals. Such was the case in the 2014 spillage of 27,000 gallons and the 2021 spillage of 14,000 gallons of fuel. Water samplings indicated an increase in toxic chemicals in the water. In one photo taken of a glass container of water drawn after 2014 one can easily see fuel floating on top of the water. Following the 2021 spill TPH-Diesel reached 4,100 ppb, the Hawaii Health Department's environmental action level (EAL) for

TPH-Diesel is 400 ppb, which had been raised from a level of 100 ppb in 2017. (Chua 2022)

Based on the long history of poorly maintained tanks, valves and, piping, the documented amounts of leaks and spills, and the high probability that leaks and spillages occurred that were never documented, it would seem likely that anyone who drank, washed in the contaminated water, or had breathe the toxic vapors is at a high risk of having serious health issues.

Should the government make an effort to notify those who were stationed or lived on the base in prior years of the contamination issues and how important health screenings are? Of course, they should!

The Sierra Club of Hawaii has clashed with the Navy for many years over contamination issues at Red Hill. In my efforts to update this manuscript to include the Red Hill tragedy, the Sierra Club of Hawaii's Wayne Tanaka has provided important and sensitive information and also computer links to such information. Truly, a most passionate group whose tireless efforts to keep the Oahu Sole Source Aquifer safe has been frustrating, inspiring and most meaningful.

One such link led me to written expert testimony provided by Dr. Nicole M. DeNovio, PHD a licensed hydrogeologist and licensed geologist. The expert testimony, dated January 19, 2021, was provided on behalf of Board of Water Supply, City and County of Honolulu during a hearing for a permit application submitted by the Navy. Included are several graphs that help reflect what has taken place.

Dr. DeNovio's expert written testimony consisted of nearly 100 pages. Her report included the statement, **"It is undisputed that these fuel releases have contaminated the environment in the Tank Farm, including the Sole Source Aquifer."**

After what occurred at Camp Lejeune how could the Navy knowingly just standby for another four decades and do so little, if anything at all, to protect the good health of so many on this beautiful island paradise of Oahu, Hawaii?

Included within Dr. DeNovio's written testimony are several graphs. Following are three and the information contained was gathered from facility histories, inspection reports, Navy release notifications and Navy witness testimony.

The first graph reflects cumulative reported fuel releases in gallons from 1940 to 2020. It is both puzzling and suspicious that when the Camp Lejeune tragedy started unfolding in the mid-1980's the fuel releases stopped occurring at Red Hill and then stopped for many years.

The second graph shows the gallons of fuel released and the number of water quality samples taken for a specific year. The Navy indicates no fuel releases from 1984 until 1998, a somewhat minor release in 1998, and not another release until 2014. From 1970 through 1983, a relatively short period of time, many thousands of gallons of fuel leaked or spilled. Water quality sampling didn't begin at Red Hill until around 1998, many years after Camp Lejeune shut down wells.

A third graph again shows the gallons of fuel released in specific years. Then through water quality water samples the fuel components that were detected in that specific year. A 2014 fuel release shows a significant spike in fuel components in that year. Also, prior years had toxic issues.

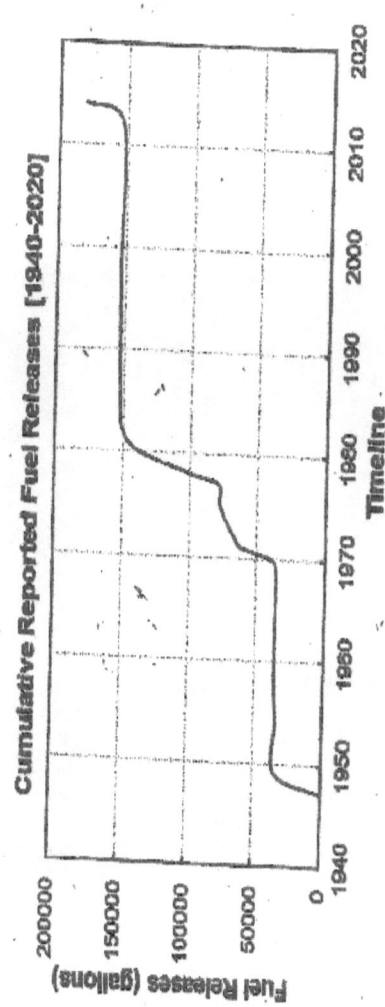

Figure 2.2-2 Cumulative fuel release volumes as reported from Facility histories, API 653 inspections, Navy release notifications, and Navy witness testimony.

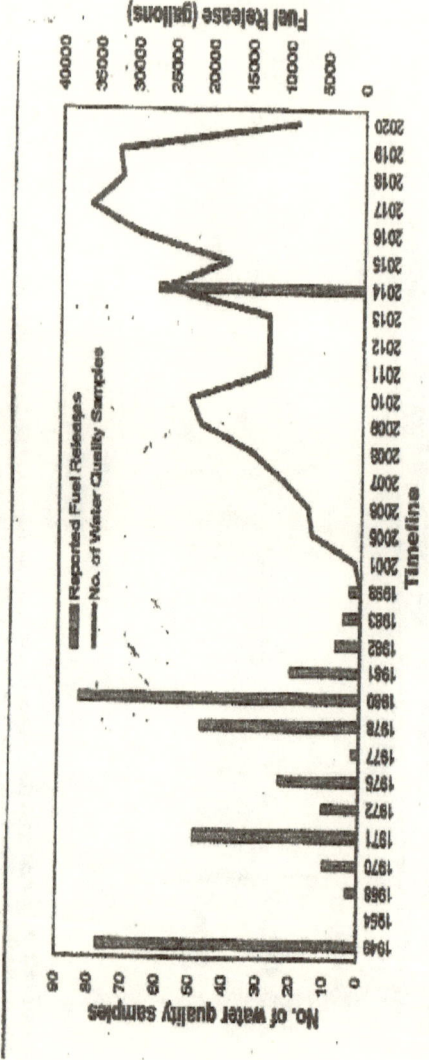

Notes: Only fuel releases with known volumes are included for reference.

Figure 2.2-3 Frequency of Water Quality Samples (1949 to March 2020)

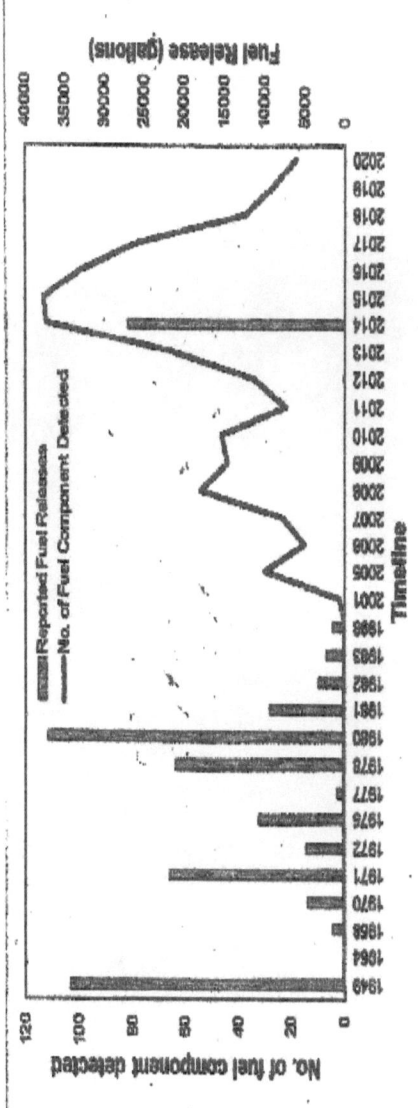

Notes: Only fuel releases with known volumes are included for reference

Figure 2.2-4 Frequency of Detected Fuel Components in Groundwater Quality Samples (1949 to March 2020)

Deadly S.N.A.F.U.

ABOUT THE AUTHOR

George Swimmer is a retired certified public accountant (CPA) who received his Bachelor of Science degree from Northern Illinois University. He is also a former registered investment advisor and has held various insurance licenses. He is a certified nursing assistant (CNA).

Swimmer served six years in the United States Marine Corps Active Reserves (1965-1971). After serving six months on active duty, he was attached to the 81MM Mortar Platoon, H & S Co., 2nd Bn., 24th Marines, 4th Marine Division headquartered in Chicago. His six months on active duty included three months at Camp Lejeune, North Carolina.

As an outspoken advocate he has spent over twenty-five years investigating train accidents and arguing for improved railroad safety. His "Railroad Collisions, A Deadly Story of Mismanaged Risk", is an acclaimed non-fiction memoir that tells of his many years of investigating train accidents and his efforts to improve railroad safety.

Swimmer is a recipient of the Citizen Advocacy Center's Citizen Initiative Award, the Lions Clubs International Foundation's Melvin Jones Fellow

Award, and the DuPage Railroad Safety Council's Jonathon Goers Award.

A former member of the Illinois Task Force on Fetal Alcohol Spectrum Disorders (FASD). The founder and former member of Illinois FACES, a foster parent advocacy group.

Please consider an Amazon review.

George Swimmer can be contacted at, <u>GeorgeSwimmer1@gmail.com</u>

APPENDIX A, VETERANS AFFAIRS ADMINISTRATION

VA Benefits

Family member health care reimbursement

Family members of Veterans who also resided at Camp Lejeune during the qualifying period are eligible for reimbursement of out-of-pocket medical expenses related to the 15 covered health conditions. VA can only pay treatment costs that remain after payment from your other health plans.

As a part of the Caring for Camp Lejeune Families Act of 2012, qualifying Veterans could receive all their health care (except dental care) from VA if they served on active duty at Camp Lejeune for at least 30 days between August 1, 1953 and December 31, 1987, even if they don't have a health condition that is presumed to be related to exposure. For individuals with one of the 15 medical conditions presumed to be related to exposure, there is no charge for care. For other health conditions, Veterans will have a co-pay, depending on income and health eligibility priority category.

Veterans' health care

Deadly S.N.A.F.U.

In accordance with the 2012 Camp Lejeune health care law, VA provides cost-free health care for certain conditions to Veterans who served at least 30 days of active duty at Camp Lejeune from August 1, 1953 and December 31, 1987.

Qualifying health conditions include:

Esophageal cancer

Breast cancer

Kidney cancer

Multiple myeloma

Renal toxicity

Female infertility

Scleroderma

Non-Hodgkin's lymphoma

Lung cancer

Bladder cancer

Leukemia

Myelodysplastic syndromes

Hepatic steatosis

Miscarriage

Neurobehavioral effects

Disability compensation

VA has established a presumptive service connection for Veterans, Reservists, and National Guard members exposed to contaminants in the water supply at Camp Lejeune from August 1, 1953 through December 31, 1987 who later developed one of the following eight diseases:

- Adult leukemia

- Aplastic anemia and other myelodysplastic syndromes

- Bladder cancer

- Kidney cancer

- Liver cancer

- Multiple myeloma

- Non-Hodgkin's lymphoma

- Parkinson's disease

Camp Lejeune Disability Benefit Coverage Area

Not yet enrolled in VA health care? **Apply online** or call 1-877-222-8387 for help.

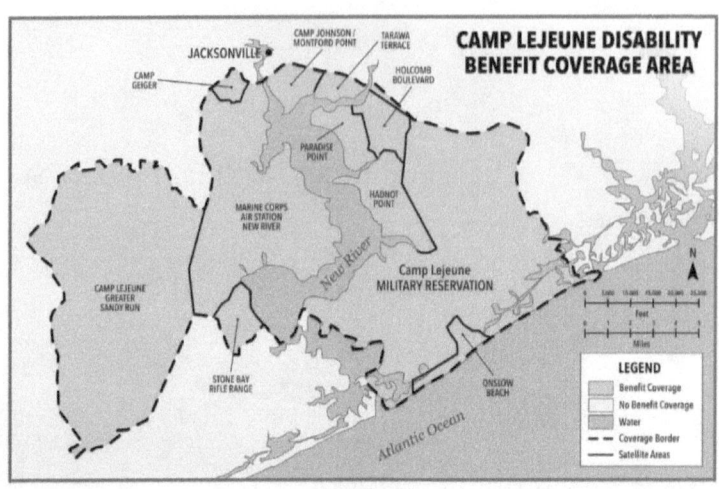

Family member health care reimbursement

Family members of Veterans who also resided at Camp Lejeune during the qualifying period are eligible for reimbursement of out-of-pocket medical expenses related to the 15 covered health conditions. VA can only pay treatment costs that remain after payment from your other health plans.

Apply online for reimbursement or call 1-866-372-1144 for help.

What type of evidence can I submit with my application?

George Swimmer

Documentation showing dependent relationship to a Veteran who served at Camp Lejeune, such as marriage license or birth certificate.

Documentation showing you lived on the base for 30 days or more between Aug. 1, 1953 and Dec. 31, 1987 such as copies of orders or base housing records.

You paid health care expenses for a covered condition respective to the following date ranges.

If you lived on Camp Lejeune between January 1, 1957 and December 31, 1987, then you can be reimbursed for care that you received on or after August 6, 2012.

If you lived on Camp Lejeune between August 1, 1953 and December 31, 1956, then you can be reimbursed for care that you received on or after December 16, 2014.

When evidence is not submitted, VA will use all relevant evidence from internal sources and the Department of Defense (DoD) to support your application. Please be aware it may take longer to review your application. **(Affairs n.d.)**

CAMP LEJEUNE FAMILY MEMBER PROGRAM

The Camp Lejeune *Family Member* Program is for *family members* of *Veterans* who were stationed at Camp Lejeune from August 1, 1953, through December 31, 1987, people living at the U.S. Marine Corps Base Camp Lejeune, North Carolina, and were potentially exposed to drinking water contaminated with industrial solvents, benzene, and other chemicals. On August 6, 2012, the Honoring America's Veterans and Caring for Camp Lejeune Families Act of 2012 was signed into law. This law (H.R. 1627, now Public Law 112-154) requires the Department of Veterans Affairs (VA) to provide health care to Veterans who served on active duty at Camp Lejeune and to reimburse eligible Camp Lejeune Family Members (CLFM) for eligible health care costs related to one or more of 15 specified illnesses or conditions illustrated in the list below.

Bladder cancer

Breast cancer

Esophageal cancer

Female infertility

Hepatic steatosis

Kidney cancer

George Swimmer

Leukemia

Lung cancer

Miscarriage

Multiple myeloma

Myelodysplastic syndromes

Neurobehavioral effects

Non-Hodgkin's lymphoma

Renal toxicity

Scleroderma

This website will assist CLFMs who want to apply for reimbursement of health care expenses related to one or more of the 15 conditions below. Please review the information on this page to assist you with applying for the Camp Lejeune Family Member Program (CLFMP). When you are ready, scroll to the bottom of this page and select "Start New Application for Family Member". If you've already started the application process, select "Retrieve Saved Application."

Please note: This program is *only* for family members of Veterans who were stationed at Camp Lejeune. If you are a Veteran, call 1-877-222-8387 for help.

Deadly S.N.A.F.U.

Frequently Asked Questions

How do I apply for the CLFM Program?

For standard processing, complete a **paper application** and fax to (512) 460-5536 *or* mail to:

Department of Veterans Affairs
Financial Services Center
PO BOX 149200
Austin, TX 78714-9200

What type of evidence do I need to submit with my application?

VA will need evidence that you were both a legal dependent of the Veteran and that you were a resident at Camp Lejeune for at least 30 days between the dates of August 1, 1953, and December 31, 1987.

What type of evidence do I need to submit? Legal dependency documents include, but are not limited to:

- marriage certificate,
- birth certificate,
- adoption papers, or

- other legal documents.

Proof of Camp Lejeune residency documents include, but are not limited to:

- military orders,

- base housing records,

- utility bill,

- pay stub,

- tax forms, or

- similar documentation.

Will the VA assist me in locating evidence?
VA will attempt to obtain all relevant evidence available for you within the Veterans Health Administration (VHA), the Veterans Benefits Administration (VBA), and the Department of Defense (DoD).
Please note: VA will still review your application if you do not send evidence, but it may take longer to process while we confirm information with other agencies.

Am I required to fill out a CLFM Treating Physician   Report?

Deadly S.N.A.F.U.

If you have one of the 15 CLFMP medical conditions, you may wish to provide a copy of the **Treating Physician Report** to your physician for completion. Submission of this form is **not** required; however, this assists us with important information to process your clinical eligibility.

For your clinical eligibility determination, Medical records must be sent in and must show:

•   The date of onset of any condition which you are claiming under this program *and*

•   That you are currently receiving treatment from your physician for this condition.

If you are not currently receiving treatment for this condition, please submit medical records that show you have received treatment in the past. The covered conditions are listed below.

Bladder cancer	Miscarriage
	Multiple myeloma
Breast cancer	Myelodysplastic syndromes
Esophageal cancer	Neurobehavioral effects
Female infertility	Non-Hodgkin's
Hepatic	

George Swimmer

steatosis	lymphoma
Kidney cancer	Renal toxicity
Leukemia	Scleroderma
Lung cancer	

What do I do if I forgot something on my application?

Contact us at: 1-866-372-1144 for assistance.

What do I do if my information needs to be updated?

Complete the <u>CLFMP Information Update Form</u> for address and health insurance changes.

APPENDIX B, DOCUMENTARY, SEMPER FIDELIS: ALWAYS FAITHFUL

This award-winning documentary is available for purchase or rental on YouTube. The film will touch an emotional nerve and almost bring you to tears, at the same time you will feel like shouting out words of anger. Water is our life source, and for the Marine Corps to allow it to be poisoned with toxic chemicals through so many years of ineptitude and neglect and then for decades not notify those of us who drank and washed in that poison is appalling.

Semper Fi: Always Faithful, is a documentary film about the Camp Lejeune water contamination. The film made the 15 film short list for consideration for a 2012 Academy Award for best documentary feature. The film won a documentary editing award at Tribeca and The Ridenhour Documentary Film Prize 2012. The Society of Professional Journalists presented it with its Sigma Delta Chi Award for Best Television Documentary.

Jerry Ensminger was a devoted Marine Corps Master Sgt. for nearly twenty-five years. As a drill instructor he lived and breathed the "Corps" and was responsible for indoctrinating thousands of new recruits with its motto Semper Fidelis or "Always

George Swimmer

Faithful." When Jerry's nine-year-old daughter Janey died of a rare type of leukemia, his world collapsed. As a grief-stricken father, he struggled for years to make sense of what happened. His search for answers led to the shocking discovery of a Marine Corps cover-up of one of the largest water contamination incidents in U.S. history. Semper Fi: Always Faithful follows Jerry's mission to expose the Marine Corps and force them to live up to their motto to the thousands of Marines and their families exposed to toxic chemicals. His fight reveals a grave injustice at North Carolina's Camp Lejeune and a looming environmental crisis at military sites across the country. (Wik)

The film has brought awareness to the importance of clean water and what will occur when a water supply system is contaminated through mismanagement. Sadly, Marine Corps Base Camp Lejeune is just one striking example of many military bases where the mismanagement of fuels and chemicals has led to an untold high number of sick and dead.

The good news is that of many of us who were not previously entitled to VA benefits, now are. The bad news is that many are still not aware of the contamination issue and the ones that are, and file for VA benefits, face an uphill battle to receive these deserved benefits.

To those who participated in the making of this documentary film or have advocated for those of us who drank and washed in contaminated water, thank you. Your efforts are heroic.

APPENDIX C, NATIONAL DEFENSE AUTHORIZATION ACT FOR FISCAL YEAR 2008

Public Law 110-181 110th Congress

SEC. 315. <<NOTE: Deadlines>> NOTIFICATION OF CERTAIN RESIDENTS AND CIVILIAN EMPLOYEES AT CAMP LEJEUNE, NORTH CAROLINA, OF EXPOSURE TO DRINKING WATER CONTAMINATION.

(a) Notification of Individuals Served by Tarawa Terrace Water Distribution System, Including Knox Trailer Park. --Not later than 1 year after the date of the enactment of this Act, the Secretary of the Navy shall make reasonable efforts to identify and notify directly individuals who were served by the Tarawa Terrace Water Distribution System, including Knox Trailer Park, at Camp Lejeune, North Carolina, during the years 1958 through 1987 that they may have been exposed to drinking water contaminated with tetrachloroethylene (PCE). (b) Notification of Individuals Served by Hadnot Point Water Distribution System. --Not later than 1 year after the Agency for Toxic Substances and Disease Registry (ATSDR) completes its water modeling study of the Hadnot Point water distribution system, the Secretary of the Navy shall make reasonable efforts to identify and notify directly individuals who were served by the system during the period identified in the study of the drinking water contamination to which they may have been exposed.

(c) Notification of Former Civilian Employees at Camp Lejeune. --Not later than 1 year after the date of the enactment

[[Page 122 STAT. 57]] of this Act, the Secretary of the Navy shall make reasonable efforts to identify and notify directly civilian employees who worked at Camp Lejeune during the period identified in the ATSDR drinking water study of the drinking water contamination to which they may have been exposed.

(d) Circulation of Health Survey. --

(1) Findings. --Congress makes the following findings:

(A) Notification and survey efforts related to the drinking water contamination described in this section are necessary due to the potential negative health impacts of these contaminants.

(B) The Secretary of the Navy will not be able to identify or contact all former residents and former employees due to the condition, non-existence, or accessibility of records.

(C) It is the intent of Congress that the Secretary of the Navy contact as many former residents and former employees as quickly as possible.

(2) ATSDR health survey. --

(A) Development. --

(i) In general. --Not later than 120 days after the date of the enactment of this Act, the ATSDR, in consultation with a well-qualified contractor selected by the ATSDR, shall develop a health survey that would voluntarily request of individuals described in subsections (a), (b), and (c) personal health information that may lead to scientifically useful health information associated with exposure to trichloroethylene (TCE), PCE, vinyl chloride, and the other contaminants identified in the ATSDR studies that may provide a basis for further reliable scientific studies of potentially adverse health impacts of exposure to contaminated water at Camp Lejeune. (ii) Funding.--The Secretary of the Navy is authorized to provide from available funds the necessary funding for the ATSDR to develop the health survey.

(B) Inclusion with notification. --The survey developed under subparagraph (A) shall be distributed by the Secretary of the Navy concurrently with the direct notification required under subsections (a), (b), and (c).

(e) Use of Media to Supplement Notification.-- The Secretary of the Navy may use media notification as a supplement to direct notification of individuals described under subsections (a), (b), and (c). Media notification may reach those individuals not identifiable via remaining records. Once individuals respond to media notifications, the Secretary will add them to the contact list to be included in future information updates.

(National Defense Authorization Act of Fiscal Year 2008 n.d.)

***

The federal law allows for media usage by the Department of the Navy to help in the notification of those *individuals not identifiable* by the Department of the Navy. This federal law comes almost thirty years after the Marine Corps first became aware of the contamination issue. The public law continues to allow the notification process to be made thru the Department of the Navy and provides them with an excuse for not directly notifying those of us who were at Camp Lejeune during the timeframe indicated. The

Marine Corps is a component of the Department of the Navy. It brings to mind the old saying "fool me once shame on you, fool me twice **shame** on me". As this manuscript continues, I will argue that many of, if not all Marine Corps Active Reservists, who had been impacted by this tragedy were never directly notified. Also, that many are still not aware of the problem or that they are now or could be entitled to VA benefits. It is my estimate that the number of Marine Corps Active Reservists who served at the base and impacted could be about 100,000. Also, many Marine regulars have still not been directly notified.

APPENDIX D, CHEMICALS AT CAMP LEJEUNE (FAQS)

1. What chemicals were found at the Tarawa Terrace Treatment Plant?

Tetrachloroethylene (also known as perchloroethylene or "PCE") was the main contaminant. The maximum level detected in drinking water was 215 parts per billion (µg/L) in February 1985. The source of contamination was ABC One-Hour Cleaners, an off-base dry-cleaning firm. The most highly contaminated wells were shut down in February 1985. Water modeling that ATSDR conducted for the Tarawa Terrace system is complete. Based on the model results, PCE concentration was estimated to have exceeded the current EPA maximum contaminant level of 5 µg/L in drinking water at the Tarawa Terrace water treatment plant for 346 months during November 1957-February 1987. Over time, PCE degrades in ground water to trichloroethylene (TCE), trans-1,2-dichloroethylene (DCE) and vinyl chloride. Levels of these chemicals in the Tarawa Terrace drinking water system were also estimated.

Benzene was also detected during the sampling of the Tarawa Terrace drinking water system in 1985. Benzene was detected at less than 2 ppb (parts per billion) which is much lower than the current U.S. standard of 5 ppb.

2. What chemicals were found at the Hadnot Point Treatment Plant?

Trichloroethylene (TCE) was the main contaminant. The maximum level detected in drinking water was 1,400 µg/L in May 1982. The current limit for TCE in drinking water is 5 µg/L. Other contaminants detected in finished water at the Hadnot Point treatment plant included DCE (trans 1,2-dichloroethylene), PCE, benzene, and vinyl chloride. DCE was detected at a maximum of 407 µg/L in January 1985. There are reported detections of benzene in the finished water at Hadnot Point in late 1985.

There were multiple sources of contamination including leaking underground storage tanks and waste disposal sites. The most highly contaminated wells were shut down by February 1985. ATSDR modeled the contamination and determined that at least one VOC exceeded its current EPA maximum contaminant level in finished water between August 1953 and January 1985.

3. What are trichloroethylene (TCE) and perchloroethylene (PCE)? What are VOCs?

TCE and PCE are chemicals that are used in dry cleaning and in cleaning metal parts of machines. VOCs are volatile organic compounds. They are a group of chemicals that generally include solvents and fuels that evaporate easily. TCE and PCE are examples of VOCs.

4. What is benzene?

Benzene is a colorless liquid with a sweet odor that evaporates into the air very quickly and dissolves slightly in water.

Some industries use benzene to make other chemicals which are used to make plastics, resins, and nylon and synthetic fibers. Benzene is also used to make some types of rubbers, lubricants, dyes, detergents, drugs, and pesticides. Natural sources of benzene include volcanoes and forest fires. Benzene is also a natural part of crude oil, gasoline, and cigarette smoke.

5. What is vinyl chloride?

Vinyl chloride (VC) is a colorless gas at room temperature. It is in liquid form if kept under high pressure or at low temperatures. VC has a mild, sweet odor and dissolves slightly in water. It is a manufactured substance that does not occur naturally. It can be formed when other substances such as trichloroethylene (TCE) and tetrachloroethylene (PCE) are broken down. VC is used to make polyvinyl chloride (PVC). PVC is used to make a variety of plastic products, including pipes, wire and cable coatings, and packaging materials. ((ATSDR) 2014)

APPENDIX E, HEALTH ISSUES

HOW CAN BENZENE AFFECT MY HEALTH?

This fact sheet answers the most frequently asked health questions (FAQs) about benzene. For more information, call the ATSDR Information Center at 1-800-232-4636. This fact sheet is one in a series of summaries about hazardous substances and their health effects. It is important you understand this information because this substance may harm you. The effects of exposure to any hazardous substance depend on the dose, the duration, how you are exposed, personal traits and habits, and whether other chemicals are present.

Highlights

Benzene is a widely used chemical formed from both natural processes and human activities. Breathing benzene can cause drowsiness, dizziness, and unconsciousness; long-term benzene exposure causes effects on the bone marrow and can cause anemia and leukemia. Benzene has been found in at least 1,000 of the 1,684 National Priority List sites identified by the Environmental Protection Agency (EPA).

What is benzene?

Benzene is a colorless liquid with a sweet odor. It evaporates into the air very quickly and dissolves slightly in water. It is highly flammable and is formed from both natural processes and human activities.

Benzene is widely used in the United States; it ranks in the top 20 chemicals for production volume. Some industries use benzene to make other chemicals which are used to make plastics, resins, nylon and other synthetic fibers. Benzene is also used to make some types of rubbers, lubricants, dyes, detergents, drugs, and pesticides. Natural sources of benzene include emissions from volcanoes and forest fires. Benzene is also a natural part of crude oil, gasoline, and cigarette smoke.

What happens to benzene when it enters the environment?

Industrial processes are the main source of benzene in the environment.

Benzene can pass into the air from water and soil.

It reacts with other chemicals in the air and breaks down within a few days.

Benzene in the air can attach to rain or snow and be carried back down to the ground.

It breaks down more slowly in water and soil and can pass through the soil into underground water.

Benzene does not build up in plants or animals.

How might I be exposed to benzene?

Outdoor air contains low levels of benzene from tobacco smoke, automobile service stations, exhaust from motor vehicles, and industrial emissions.

Vapors (or gases) from products that contain benzene, such as glues, paints, furniture wax, and detergents, can also be a source of exposure.

Air around hazardous waste sites or gas stations will contain higher levels of benzene.

Working in industries that make or use benzene.

How can benzene affect my health?

Breathing very high levels of benzene can result in death, while high levels can cause drowsiness, dizziness, rapid heart rate, headaches, tremors, confusion, and unconsciousness. Eating or drinking foods containing high levels of benzene can cause vomiting, irritation of the stomach, dizziness, sleepiness, convulsions, rapid heart rate, and death.

175

The major effect of benzene from long-term exposure is on the blood. Benzene causes harmful effects on the bone marrow and can cause a decrease in red blood cells leading to anemia. It can also cause excessive bleeding and can affect the immune system, increasing the chance for infection.

Some women who breathed high levels of benzene for many months had irregular menstrual periods and a decrease in the size of their ovaries, but we do not know for certain that benzene caused the effects. It is not known whether benzene will affect fertility in men.

How likely is benzene to cause cancer?

Long-term exposure to high levels of benzene in the air can cause leukemia, particularly acute myelogenous leukemia, often referred to as AML. This is a cancer of the blood forming organs. The Department of Health and Human Services (DHHS) has determined that benzene is a known carcinogen. The International Agency for Research on Cancer (IARC) and the EPA have determined that benzene is carcinogenic to humans.

How can benzene affect children?

Children can be affected by benzene exposure in the same ways as adults. It is not known if children are more susceptible to benzene poisoning than adults.

Benzene can pass from the mother's blood to a fetus. Animal studies have shown low birth weights, delayed bone formation, and bone marrow damage when pregnant animals breathed benzene.

How can families reduce the risks of exposure to benzene?

Benzene exposure can be reduced by limiting contact with gasoline and cigarette smoke. Families are encouraged not to smoke in their house, in enclosed environments, or near their children.

Is there a medical test to show whether I've been exposed to benzene?

Several tests can show if you have been exposed to benzene. There is a test for measuring benzene in the breath; this test must be done shortly after exposure. Benzene can also be measured in the blood; however, since benzene disappears rapidly from the blood, this test is only useful for recent exposures.

In the body, benzene is converted to products called metabolites. Certain metabolites can be measured in the urine. The metabolite S-phenylmercapturic acid in urine is a sensitive indicator of benzene exposure. However, this test must be done shortly after exposure and is not a reliable indicator of how much benzene you have been exposed to, since the metabolites may be present in urine from other sources.

Has the federal government made recommendations to protect human health?

The EPA has set the maximum permissible level of benzene in drinking water at 5 parts benzene per billion parts of water (5 ppb).

The Occupational Safety and Health Administration (OSHA) has set limits of 1-part benzene per million parts of workplace air (1 ppm) for 8 hour shifts and 40-hour work weeks.

References

Agency for Toxic Substances and Disease Registry (ATSDR). 2007. Toxicological Profile for Benzene *(Update)*. Atlanta, GA: U.S. Department of Health and Human Services, Public Health Service.

Where can I get more information?

If you have questions or concerns, please contact your community or state health or environmental quality department or:

For more information, contact:
Agency for Toxic Substances and Disease Registry
Division of Toxicology and Human Health Sciences

1600 Clifton Road NE, Mailstop S102-1
Atlanta, GA 30333
Phone: 1-800-CDC-INFO · 888-232-6348 (TTY)
Email: Contact CDC-INFO

ATSDR can also tell you the location of occupational and environmental health clinics. These clinics specialize in recognizing, evaluating, and treating illnesses resulting from exposure to hazardous substances. (TaxFAQ for Benzene updated 2015)

There was one time when I became so sick at Camp Lejeune that I went to sick bay and was laying on a bench in horrible pain. Someone in charge came in and told me to sit up. He then asked, do you think you are dying? When I said yes and I meant it, I received immediate attention. I stayed in sick bay a day or two, recovered and went back to my platoon. Looking back, I suspect that I had some type of poisoning.

TRICHLOROETHYLENE (TCE)

Affected Organ Systems: Developmental (effects during periods when organs are developing), Neurological (Nervous System)

Cancer Classification: EPA: Carcinogenic to humans, IARC: Carcinogenic to humans (evidence for cancer is based on kidney cancer, limited evidence for non-Hodgkin lymphoma and liver cancer, as well as various tumors in animals). NTP: Known to be a Human Carcinogen.

Please contact NTP, IARC, or EPA's IRIS Hotline with questions on cancer and cancer classification.

Chemical Classification: Volatile organic compounds

Summary: Trichloroethylene (TCE) is a nonflammable, colorless liquid with a somewhat sweet odor and a sweet, burning taste. It is used mainly as a solvent to remove grease from metal parts, but it is also an ingredient in adhesives, paint removers, typewriter correction fluids, and spot removers. Trichloroethylene is not thought to occur naturally in the environment. However, it has been found in underground water sources and many surface waters as a result of the manufacture, use, and disposal of the chemical. (Registry n.d.)

PERCHLOROETHYLENE (PCE)

Synonyms: perchloroethene, tetrachloroethene, tetrachloroethylene, may also be referred to as "Perc"

PCE is an **organic chemical** introduced in the environment by human activity. Specifically, it is a widely used solvent, especially in dry cleaning activities. PCE is also used as a degreaser and in some consumer products (e.g., shoe polish, typewriter correction fluid). Although not theoretically impossible, there is no evidence that PCE forms or occurs naturally in the environment. Thus, its detection in an environmental sample (e.g., groundwater, surface water, soil, indoor, or ambient air) is associated with PCE spills or accidental release.

PCE is toxic to humans at very low concentrations. The Environmental Protection Agency has established a Maximum Contaminant Level for PCE in water of 5 parts per billion (or micrograms per Liter). At this low amount, practically PCE cannot be perceived by smell or taste. For example, people may smell PCE in air at concentrations above 1 ppm (parts per million).

Where Is PCE Used/Found?

- dry cleaning / dry cleaned clothes
- degreasing activities / industrial sites

consumer products (e.g., shoe polish, typewriter correction fluid)

- manufacturing and auto repair shops

- manufacturing of chlorofluorocarbons

- auto paint

- electroplating

- General Description/Properties

PCE is a **halogenated organic** compound composed of 2 atoms of carbon and 4 atoms of chlorine (two chlorine atoms linked to each carbon). The two carbons are linked with each other by a double chemical bond. Thus, PCE does not contain any hydrogen atoms.

PCE is a colorless liquid with a sweetish smell which is not flammable under normal temperature and pressure. It is part of a class of chemicals also known as halogenated volatile organic compounds (HVOCs). This means that PCE evaporates (goes from liquid into gaseous form when in contact with air).

PCE is also part of a class of chemicals referred to as "chlorinated solvents". Due to the presence of one or more chlorine atoms in their structure chlorinated solvents are heavier than water. Chlorinated solvents are also referred to as Dense Non-Aqueous Phase Liquids (DNAPLs).

Environment Fate and Transport: Basically, when spilled into the environment, part of the spilled PCE will evaporate, while another part will infiltrate through the ground into the subsurface.

- **Air**: Once in air, PCE was shown to be oxidized with a half-life of 96 days.

- **Subsurface**: Once in the subsurface, PCE will move downward under the influence of gravity. Its downward movement will be slowed down or sometimes even stopped by layers of low permeability (such as clays or silts). When this happens, PCE will start moving laterally following the slope of the low permeability layer until it either reaches a dip in the layer and accumulates in pools or until it finds a hole in the layer which enables further downward movement. Usually, groundwater will also sit on less permeable subsurface layers thus the subsurface accumulated pools of PCE will serve as a secondary source providing PCE into water continuously until the PCE underground accumulated pool gets depleted.

- **Groundwater**: When it comes in contact with groundwater, PCE will start dissolving in groundwater until it reaches its solubility limit. Thus, when in contact with groundwater part of PCE will solubilize and the remaining part will continue to travel downward percolating the water table and accumulating at the bottom of the water since PCE is heavier (more dense) than water. The PCE sitting on the bottom of water will act as a secondary source by continuously dissolving PCE into the water.

Thus, PCE may travel in the subsurface as a DNAPL, as a dissolved phase into groundwater, and as a gaseous phase. As a DNAPL, PCE may accumulate on the bottom of groundwater table in a dip. DNAPL flow direction is in general independent from groundwater flow direction, as it relates to sloping of underground low permeable layers. In contrast, the dissolved PCE phase will travel with groundwater. During subsurface transport, some PCE may be absorbed to soil particles.

What makes PCE a problematic pollutant is its resistance to degradation/biodegradation, unlike, petroleum hydrocarbons (which usually degrade fast in the environment). How Can You Be Exposed to PCE?

Through inhalation:

- breathing in air contaminated with gaseous PCE:
  -             indoor air from a building sitting on contaminated

              soil and/or groundwater
  -             indoor air from a workplace where PCE is

manufactured or used (e.g., in dry cleaning)

- breathing the PCE vapors during a bath or shower with contaminated water (especially when well water and not municipal water is used)
- wearing dry cleaned clothes soon after they are dry cleaned
- breathing in the vicinity of a person who was recently exposed to PCE (e.g., workers) - such person may exhale PCE vapors

Through skin absorption (please note that PCE is not efficiently absorbed through the skin):

- Playing on contaminated ground

- Bathing in contaminated water

Spending time in a contaminated atmosphere

wearing dry cleaned clothes soon after they are dry cleaned

Through ingestion:

- Contaminated water

- Contaminated food

- Accidentally ingest contaminated particles (e.g., soil)

Through breast feeding – since PCE accumulates in milk due to its lipophilic nature,

Non-Cancer Effects

Exposure to PCE may cause a variety of health effects depending on the amount of PCE and exposure time. Such effects may include:

In chronic exposures:

- Skin irritation

- Dizziness

- Headache

- Liver and kidney damage

Menstrual problems and spontaneous abortions (in exposed women)

In acute exposures (to high amounts of PCE):

Central nervous system damage (for exposure to more than 100 ppm pf PCE):
- Unconsciousness
- Difficulty in walking and speaking
- Nausea
- Vomiting

- Death from respiratory depression (ingestion of more than 1,500 ppm of PCE)

- Death (within 4 hours) – by ingestion of 2,600-4,000 ppm PCE (experiments with rats)

Please note that the data related to such **exposure pollution** is usually obtained through animal studies and may not be verified in humans, however the potential to cause similar problems in humans remains.

Cancer Effects

PCE is reasonably anticipated carcinogen, which means that it was proven to cause tumors in mice, and it has the potential to cause cancer in humans, especially when exposure to high amounts of PCE has occurred. The following type of cancers may be associated to exposure to PCE:

Lung cancer, Cancer of colon-rectum, Esophageal cancer, Bladder cancer

(Centers n.d.)

OUR IMMUNE SYSTEM

Some chemicals cause damage to the immune system and become detectable only after a long period of existing but not yet developed or manifested. Some exposure to chemicals, often synthetic chemicals, can present additional risk to individuals with an immune system that is already fragile; for example, people who already have a primary immune deficiency, or infants or persons of old age.

Some groups of individuals exposed to environmental contaminants could be at greater risk of damage to their immune system. With an unborn child, when the immune system is developing, the damage to the immune system could have long term effects on the ability of an individual to generate an adequate immune response. Infants and young people also are at increased risk from environmental toxicants in that childhood is the time when primary immunity is often developed. As a person ages their immune system begins to decline. Because the immune function declines as a person ages there is an increase in the incidence of tumors.

Other factors that can prevent or inhibit the immune system from working effectively are smoking, diet, malnutrition, stress and disease. Some chemical diseases damage the immune system and become detectable only after a long period of existing but have not yet developed or manifested. (Immunotoxicology 1992)

Deadly S.N.A.F.U.

HEALTH CONCERNS AT CAMP LEJEUNE

ATSDR is concerned about the health effects of exposures to chemicals found in the drinking water at Camp Lejeune. Before 1986, drinking water from the Tarawa Terrace and Hadnot Point treatment plants were contaminated with volatile organic compounds (VOCs). The main VOC found at Tarawa Terrace was perchloroethylene (PCE). The maximum level of PCE found in the Tarawa Terrace drinking water system was 215 micrograms per liter (µg/L), which was 43 times higher than the current U.S. maximum contaminant level (MCL) allowed in drinking water of 5 µg/L. The VOCs found at Hadnot Point were trichloroethylene (TCE), vinyl chloride, benzene, and trans-1,2-dichloroethylene (DCE). The maximum level of TCE found in the Hadnot Point drinking water system was 1,400 µg/L which was 280 times higher than the current U.S. maximum contaminant level (MCL) allowed in drinking water of 5 µg/L.

TCE, vinyl chloride, and benzene are classified as human carcinogens, while PCE is classified as a "likely" or "probable" human carcinogen (1-6). The carcinogenicity of DCE cannot be classified because of a lack of studies.

George Swimmer

Former Marines, Employees, and Dependents Potentially Exposed to Contaminated Drinking Water at USMC Base Camp Lejeune: A Summary of Agency for Toxic Substances and Disease Registry (ATSDR) Study Design and Results

Study Purpose

Some residents and civilian employees who lived or worked at Camp Lejeune from the 1950s through 1985 were exposed to drinking water contaminated with volatile organic compounds. The purpose of this study was to determine whether there is a link between exposure to contaminated drinking water at Camp Lejeune and selected cancers or other diseases in former service men and women, their families, and civilian workers.
Drinking water at Camp Lejeune was contaminated with volatile organic compounds (VOCs), including trichloroethylene (TCE), tetrachloroethylene (PCE), benzene, trans-1,2-dichloroethylene (DCE), and vinyl chloride.

What Was Studied

Health surveys were mailed to over 247,000 study participants or their next of kin. Over 76,000 surveys were completed, collecting information about cancers and other diseases, including type of disease and age of diagnosis, as well as factors that affect health like age, race, education, smoking, and alcohol use.

Features of this Study.

This study looked at military personnel, their families, and civilian employees at Camp Lejeune who may have been exposed to contaminated drinking water and compared some specific health problems with military personnel and civilian employees at Camp Pendleton who were not exposed to the water. Using a comparison group with a similar population who was not exposed helps assess if there is a link between exposure to the water and diseases. In addition, the researchers conducted an 'internal' analyses (looking at the exposed populations within Camp Lejeune only) to see if increasing levels of exposure to the contaminants in the drinking water resulted in increased risk of disease.

Conclusion and Key Results

This study shows that contaminated drinking water at Camp Lejeune was linked to increased risk for bladder cancer, kidney cancer, and kidney disease.

Exposure to both TCE and PCE was associated with an increased risk for kidney cancer in both Marines and civilian employees.

Exposure to both TCE and PCE was associated with increased risk for bladder cancer and kidney disease in civilian employees.

Exposure to PCE was associated with increased risk for bladder cancer and kidney disease in Marines.

Risk increased with increasing levels of exposure to the contaminants for kidney cancer (TCE and PCE in Marines and TCE/PCE in civilian employees) and kidney disease (PCE in Marines and TCE/PCE in civilian employees).
These results are consistent with results found in previous studies. (Registry n.d.)

Deadly S.N.A.F.U.

ADVERSE BIRTH OUTCOMES STUDY RESULTS

Evaluation of contaminated drinking water and preterm birth, small for gestational age, and birth weight at Marine Corps Base Camp Lejeune, North Carolina: A cross-sectional study

Study Purpose

The purpose of this study was to determine if maternal exposures to contaminants in drinking water at Camp Lejeune were associated with preterm birth and fetal growth retardation. This study is a reanalysis of a previous study, which incorrectly categorized as "unexposed" some maternal exposures before June 1972 based on information available at the time.

Besides considering the re-categorized births to exposed women, the Agency for Toxic Substances and Disease Registry (ATSDR) recreated monthly estimates of past levels of drinking water contamination using computer models. These estimates were not available when the first study was conducted.

Drinking water at Camp Lejeune was contaminated with volatile organic compounds (VOCs) including trichloroethylene (TCE), tetrachloroethylene (PCE), benzene, 1,2-dichloroethylene (DCE) and vinyl chloride from the 1950s through 1985.

What Was Studied

The study included live singleton births 28-47 weeks gestation weighing 500 grams or more. The births occurred between 1968 and 1985 to women who resided on base for at least one week before giving birth. These years were chosen because computerized birth certificates in North Carolina became available in 1968 and the contaminated wells on base were shut down in 1985. The authors cross referenced birth certificate data for Onslow County, NC, where Camp Lejeune is located, with Camp Lejeune housing records and identified 11,896 births that met the study criteria.

Outcomes of interest in this study were preterm birth and fetal growth retardation. Fetal growth retardation was measured by reduced mean birth weight (MBW), term low birth weight (TLBW), and small for gestational age (SGA). Information about these outcomes was obtained from birth certificates. Preterm births were defined as births occurring at less than 37 weeks of gestation. Gestational age was calculated using date of mother's last menstrual period from the birth certificate. TLBW was defined as full-term babies (37 weeks or more gestation) weighing less than 2,500 grams at birth. SGA births were defined as births weighing less than the 10th percentiles using sex- and race-specific weight by gestational week norms. For the MBW analysis, only full-term infants were included.

Features of this Study.

Because of the lack of exposure information, ATSDR used extensive water modeling to reconstruct exposures before 1987. The water modeling allowed the investigators to examine associations between monthly estimates of exposures to VOCs in drinking water at the residences and the risk of adverse birth outcomes.

Conclusion and Key Results

The following effects were seen in births from 1968-1985 to women exposed to contaminated drinking water at Camp Lejeune. These findings also apply to women who gave birth before 1968 if they were exposed to similar levels of VOCs-contaminated drinking water.

Exposure to PCE in the womb was associated with preterm birth (before 37 weeks of pregnancy).

For PCE and preterm birth, the strongest association was seen for exposures during the 2nd trimester (4th to 6th months).

Exposure to TCE in the womb was associated with SGA, TLBW and reduced MBW.

The risk of TLBW increased with increasing levels of exposure to TCE during the 2nd trimester.

The finding for SGA is consistent with findings from a previous study conducted in Woburn, MA.

Exposure to benzene in the womb was associated with TLBW.

The risk of TLBW increased with increasing levels of exposure to benzene throughout the pregnancy. (Registry n.d.)

APPENDIX F, PFAS

MANY MORE MILITARY BASES WITH CONTAMINATED WATER

Toxic perfluorinated chemicals known as PFAS have contaminated the drinking and washing water at hundreds of U.S. military bases. The Department of Defense has released data showing more than 600 military sites and surrounding communities were contaminated with PFAS. PFAS are manmade chemicals that once released into the environment do not break down and because of this are known as forever chemicals. PFAS from contaminated water will build up in our blood and organs and are linked to birth defects, cancers, infertility, liver damage and reduced immune responses in children. Military bases used firefighting foam that contained PFAS and the foam seeped into the groundwater. The Department of Defense has released data showing more than 600 military sites and surrounding communities were contaminated with PFAS. (EWG 2020)

PFAS COULD CONTAMINATE MORE THAN 600 MILITARY INSTALLATIONS (LISTED)

Bethel AAOF

Nome AAOF

Fort Wainwright - Gerstle River Test Site

Fort Wainwright - Haines Pipeline Facilities

Bryant Airfield- JBER

Juneau AAOF

Anniston Army Depot

Redstone Arsenal

AASF #1 R W Shepherd Hope Hull

AASF #2 Birmingham

AASF #3 Bates Field Mobile

Fort McClellan

Pelham Range

Pine Bluff Arsenal

Camp Robinson

Florence Military Reservation

Fort Huachuca

Papago Military Reservation

Presidio of Monterey

Deadly S.N.A.F.U.

Fort Hunter Liggett - Parks RFTA

Presidio of Monterey - Sharpe Army Depot

Sierra Army Depot

Military Ocean Terminal Concord

Fresno TASMG

Camp San Luis Obispo

Roseville Armory

Stockton AASF

DFSP Norwalk

DFSP Ozol

DFSP San Pedro

Moffett Field NAS

AZUSA CA NCCOSC MORRIS DA

Pueblo Army Depot

Rocky Mountain Arsenal (Commerce City)

Buckley Air Force Base AASF

Gypsum (HAATS)

Groton AVCRAD and TASMG Hangar 2

Windsor Locks AASF

River Road Training Site

Stern Armory

Wilmington Armory

George Swimmer

Duncan Armory AASF

Camp Blanding

Dade City Readiness Center

Fort Pierce Readiness Center

Lakeland Readiness Center

Mariana Readiness Center

Pensacola (Ellyson Field)

Plant City Readiness Center

Brooksville RC, AASF #2

Jacksonville, Cecil Field, AASF #1

CID CORRY STATION

Fort Benning

Georgia Garrison Training Center

Fort Gordon

Fort Gordon - Gillem Annex

Fort Stewart - Hunter AAF

General Lucius D. Clay National Guard Center

Winder Barrow County Airport (enclave)

ALBANY GA MCLB

Fort Ruger

Hilo AASF #2

USAG HI- Dillingham Military Reservation

Deadly S.N.A.F.U.

USAG HI - Fort Shafter/Tripler Army Medical Center

USAG HI – Hawaii Wheeler Army Airfield

USAG HI - Helemano RAD REC Station

USAG HI - Kahuku Training Area

USAG HI - Kilauea Military Reservation

USAG HI - Kipapa Ammunition Storage Site

USAG HI - Kunia Field Station

USAG HI - Makua Military Reservation

USAG HI – Oahu-Schofield Barracks

USAG HI - Pohakuloa Training Center

USAG HI - Waikakalaua Ammunition Storage Tunnels

Waiawa Unit Training Equipment Site (UTES)

Kalaoloa Facility (Former Barbers Point-NAS)

NAVFAC HAWAII P HARBOR

Camp Dodge Johnston Training Site

Iowa Army Ammunition Plant

Boone AASF

Davenport AASF

Waterloo Big Rock AASF #2

Edgemeade TS Mountain Home

Gowen Field Boise/Airport Training Area

Orchard MATES Boise

George Swimmer

Savanna Army Depot

Rock Island Arsenal

Chicago (Midway Armory, AASF #2)

Decatur AASF #1

Kankakee AASF / Readiness Center

Peoria AASF #3 and AASF #4

Gary AASF

Indianapolis

Salina AASF #2

Fort Riley

Topeka Forbes Field AASF #1

Blue Grass Army Depot

Boone National Guard Center - AASF

W.H. Ford Regional Training Center

Hammond AASF #1

Fort Polk

Fort Polk - Peason Ridge

Camp Beauregard

Camp Villere

Esler Field AASF #2

Devens Reserve Forces Training Area

Natick Soldier Systems Center

Camp Edwards

Westfield/Barnes AASF

Forest Glen Annex

Fort Detrick

Weide AASF (enclave on APG)

Fort Meade - Phoenix Military Reservation

NAVSURFWARCEN WBETH DD

ST INIGOES MD NAVELEXSYS

Presque Isle SFRO

Brunswick West

Brunswick East

Caswell Training Site

MTC-H Camp Grayling-Cantonment

MTC-H Camp Grayling-MATES

Grand Ledge AASF

Belmont Armory

Detroit Arsenal

Ft Custer

Lansing Airport Hangar

Camp Ripley (Installation Wide PA) (Western AOI SI)

St Cloud AASF

Camp Ripley (Eastern AOIs -SI Pa, counted on Installation wide)

George Swimmer

Holman Field AASF

Lake Camp Ripley (Eastern AOIs -SI, PA, counted on

City Ammunition Plant

Fort Leonard Wood

Jefferson City AASF/Armory

Springfield AVCRAD

Whiteman Flight Facility

KANSAS CITY MO

AASF Jackson

AASF Tupelo

AASF Meridian

Camp McCain

Camp Shelby

TASMG Gulfport

Camp Mackall

Military Ocean Terminal Sunny Point

Morrisville AASF #1

Salisbury AASF #2

Bismarck AASF Complex

Fargo AASF #2

Grand Island AASF/RC

Lincoln AASF/Readiness Center

Deadly S.N.A.F.U.

Norfolk FMS #7

AASF Concord

Stafford TS - New Hampshire TS

DFSP Newington

Picatinny Arsenal

AASF Main Hangar-cold storage

Rio Rancho

Roswell

Santa Fe AASF

White Sands Missile Range

Hawthorne Army Depot

Las Vegas Cheyenne AASF

Reno AASF

Fort Hamilton

West Point

Camp Smith/CSMS A - PA

Watervliet Arsenal

DFSP Verona

Mansfield LAHM Fire Station

Lima Army Tank Plant

Green Armory AASF#1

Rickenbacker (MTA) - AASF #2

George Swimmer

McAlester Army Ammunition Plant

Lexington AASF #1

Tulsa AASF #2

Bend COTEF (Youth Challenge)

Central Oregon Unit Training Equipment Site

Christmas Valley Radar Site

McNary Field Salem AASF

Pang Base Enclave

Biak Training Areas Brett Hall

Camp Adair Corvallis

MTA Camp Rilea

Pendleton Complex Armory / AASF

Umatilla Depot

Fort Indiantown Gap

Carlisle Barracks

Tobyhanna Army Depot

  Scranton Army Ammunition Plant

MECHANICSBURG PA NAVICP

North Smithfield

Quonset Point-AASF

Allendale Armory

McCrady Training Site

Deadly S.N.A.F.U.

Joint Forces Headquarters

Rapid City Airport Complex

Holston Army Ammunition Plant

Milan Army Ammunition Plant

AASF #2

El Campo

Red River Army Depot

Fort Hood

Fort Bliss

Ellington Field

Sustained Airborne TNG FAC

Wendover Airport - AVFAC

Dugway Proving Ground

Tooele Army Depot

Tooele Army Depot South (Deseret Chemical Depot)

White Sands Missile Range - Green River Test Site

AASF-E.J. Garn Aviation Complex

AASF Byrd Field

Chesterfield Limited AASF

Radford Army Ammunition Plant

Fort AP Hill

Ft. Belvoir AASF

George Swimmer

Fort Belvoir

JB Myer Henderson Hall

Vint Hill Farms

CHESAPEAKE VA NSGA NW

NORFOLK VA FISC

WILLIAMSBURG VA FISC CA

JFHQ Camp Johnson

South Burlington AASF / Readiness Center

AASF #2

Bremerton

Camp Murray

BREMERTON WA NAVBASE

BREMERTON PUGTSND WA FISC

INDIAN ISLAND WA NAVMAG

Badger AAP

Madison AASF #2

West Bend AASF #1 / Armory

Fixed wing AAS

CTC Camp Dawson-Kingwood

Parkersburg AASF #1

Wheeling - AASF #2

Cheyenne AASF

MEANING OF ABBREVIATIONS

Agency for Toxic Substances and Disease Registry (ATSDR)

Camp Lejeune Family Members (CLFM)

Community Assistant Panel (CAP)

Department of Defense (DoD)

Department of Veterans Affairs (VA)

Environmental Protection Agency (EPA)

Freedom of Information Act (FOIA)

National Toxicology Program (NTP)

Navy's Atlantic Division (LandDiv)

perchloroethylene or (PCE)

Public Health Assessment (PHA)

Safe Drinking Water Act (SDWA)

tetrachloroethylene--also known as

trichloroethylene (TCE)

Veterans   Benefits   Administration   (VBA)

BIBLIOGRAPHY

(ATSDR), Agency for Toxic Substances and Disease Registry. 2014.

n.d.

Affairs, U.S. Department of Veterans. n.d. "Public Health." *Camp Lejeune, Past Water Contmination,* https://www.publichealth.va.gov/exposures/camp-lejeune/.

Alex Horton, Karoun Demirjlan. 2021. "Miltiary families talk of Pearl Harbor's water ills." *The Washington Post,* December.

Anne C. Fergusion-Smith, Mary-Elizabeth Patti. 2011. "You Are What Your Dad Ate." *Science Direct,* February 2: 115-117.

ATSDR. 2020. *Vapor Intrusion Public Health Asssessment.* ATSDR.

Barrett, Barbara. 2010. "Warnings About Lejeune's Tainted Water Unheeded for Years." *Common Dreamsm McClatchy Newspapers,* April 18.

—. 2009. "Lejeune water probe: Did Marine Corps hide benzene data?" *McClatchy Newspapers,* March 9.

—. 2010. "Warnings About Lejeune's tainted water unheeded for years." *McClatchy Newspapers,* April 18.

Barrett, Franco Ordonez aand Barbara. 2012. "Obama signs law giving health care to Lejeune tainted water victims." August 6.

BenZvi, Maggie. 2022. "Navy Says Operator Error..." *Black Rifle.*

n.d. "BMJ Best Practices."

January 15, 2015. "Camp Lejeune Community Assistance Panel (CAP) Meeting." U.S. Dept of Health and Human Services, Agency for Toxic Substances and Disease Registry.

December 5, 2017. "Camp Lejeune MCB." *ProPublica.*

Centers, Environmental Pollution. n.d.

n.d. "Chemocare.com."

Chua, Anna. 2022. "Sierra Club of Hawaii."

2009. *Contaminated Water Supplies at Camp Lejeune.* The National
Academies Press: www.nap.edu, Washington, D.C.: National
Research Council of the National Academies.

Copp, Tara. 2019. "What will the Navy's denial of Camp Lejeune claims
mean for other contaminated bases?" *Your Military*, January 25.

Courtney Kube, Allen Breed. 2019. "Navy to deny all civil claims
...Lejeune water contamination." *NBC, Military*, January 24.

DeNovio, Nicole M. 2021. *Written Testimony re. Red Hill*. Dept of Health
Hawaii.

Dertouzos, John. 2009. *The Cost Effectiveness of Military Advertising.*
Prepared for The Office of The Secretary of Defense, Rand
National Defense Institute.

Environmental Science and Engineering, Inc. 1985. *Evaluation of Data
From First Round of Verification Sample Collection and Analysis,
Marine Corps Base Camp Lejeune, N.C.* Naval Facilities
Engineering Command Atlantic Division.

Eschner, Kat. 2016. "The Story of the Real Canary in the Coal Mine."
smithsonianmag.com, December 30.

EWG, contact Alex Formuzis (202) 667-6982. 2020. "PFAS Could
Contaminate More Than 600 Military Installations, DOD says."
March 16.

Faith Abubey,Lindsey Basye 201 "Most claims are being denied, some
close to death." *11Alive*, Swptember 23.

Feitshans, Ilise L. 1989. "Law and Regulations of Benzene." In
Environmantal Health Perspectives, 229-307.

Francis, Taylor &. 2014. "Fathers drinking: Also responsible for fetal
disorders?" *Science Daily*, February 14.

Gonzalez, Angi. 2022. "Navy apologizies..." *Spectrum News.*

Guide, My Base. 2018. *Joint Base Pearl Habor-Hickam.* Naval Construction Bn Cntr Gulfpor.

Health, Connecticut Dept. of Public. 2012. "Vapor Intrusion of VOC's ." Environmental Health Technical Brief.

Hearing Serial # 111-108, Subcommittee on Investigations and Oversight. 2010. *Camp Lejeune: Contamination and Compensation, Looking Back, Moving Forward.* Wshington, D.C.: Committee on Science, and Technology House of Representatives.

III, Leo Shane. 2017. "VA finalizes disability benefit plans for contaminated water at Camp Lejeune." *Pentagon & Congress,* March 14.

Immunotoxicology, Subcommittee on. 1992. *Biologic Markers in Immunotoxicology.* Washington, DC: National Acadermies Press (US)).

Jedra, Christina. 2021. "Amid 'politcal concerns' Navy kept quiet..." *Civil Beat.*

—. 2021. "How The Red Hill...Threatened Oahu's Drinking water." *Civil Beat,* December 12.

Jedra, Christina. 2022. "Consultant: Fixing Red Hill's Decrepit Infrastructure..." *Civil Beat.*

Jedra, Christina. 2021. "Whistleblower says Navy gave false testimony..." *Civil Beat.*

Jerry Ensminger, Jim Fontella, Mike Partain. n.d. *MCBCL chronology of significant events concerning VI at Hadnot Point Industrial Area.* www.TFTPTF.com.

Jonathan Day, Soham Savani, Benjamin D. Krempley, Matthew Nguyen, Joanna B. Kitlinska. 2016. "Influence of paternal preconception exposures on their offspring: through epigenetics and phenotype." *Am J Stem Cells,* May 30.

Jowers, Karen. 2021. ""I regret I did not tell..."." *Military Times.*

Jowers, Karen. 2022. "CDC wants to hear..." *Military Times.*

Jowers, Karen. 2022. "Navy cites "operator error'..." *Military Times.*

Kay, Amanda Wilcox and Lindell. 2012. "Camp Lejeune water contamination victim speaks out." *The Daily News, Jacksonville, N.C.,* September 2.

Levesque, William R.2011.Marine Corps Records on Camp Lejeune Site Missing." *The Ledger, St. Petersburg Times*, May 21.

Levesque, William R. 2009. "Camp Lejeune Water Contamination History." *St. Petersburg Times*, October 18.

n.d. "Mayo Clinic."

n.d. "Medlineplus.gov."

n.d.National Defense Authorization Act of Fiscal Year 2008. Public Law 110-181 110th Congress.

n.d. "National Kidney Foundation."

Press, The Associated. 2010. "Chemical Omitted from Lejeune Water Report." February 18.

Registry, Agency for Toxic Substances and Disease. n.d.

Registry, Agency for Toxic Substances and Disease. Jan 2017, updated. "Camp Lejeune, North Carolina."

Registry, Agency for Toxic Substances and Disease. April 2018. "Morbidity Study of Former Marines, Employees, and Dependents Potentially Exposed to Contaminated Drinking Water at U.S. Marine Corps Base Camp Lejeune."

Registry, Agency for Toxic Substances and Disease. Aug 2007 "Public Health Statement for Benzene (benceno)."

Report, Commandant Marine Corps Independent Panel's. 2004. "Camp Lejeune Water Contamination Drinking Water Fact Finding Report."

Richardson, Mahealani. 2022. "Fired Navy captain privately raised concerns..." *Hawaii News Now.*

Richardson, Mahealani. 2022. "State show "disturbing" ...plume maps." *Hawaii New Now.*

Sarvana, Adam. 2009. "The Pentagon's War on America, The Marines." *Environmental Health News,* June 26.

Schmidt, Charles W. 2018. "Chips off the Old Block: How a Father's Preconception Exposures Might Affect the Health of His Children." *Environmental Health Perspectives,* February.

School, Yale Law. 2018. "VA Defies Court Orders to Release Documents Sought by Poisoned Veterans." *Yale Law School,* February 28.

Sorg, Lisa. 2020. "A Superfund cleanup in Jacksonville failed. Without federal funding for a fix, contamination is spreading." *NC Policy Watch,* February 21.

updated 2015. *TaxFAQ for Benzene .* CAS 71-43-2, Agency for Toxic Substances and Disease Registry.

Transcript, Hearing June 12, 2007. 2007. "Poisoned Patriots: Contaminated Drinking Water at Camp Lejeune, m." Edited by Subcommittee on Oversight and Investigations House of Representative. Committee on Energy and Commerce.

Twedell, Kelly. 2013. "Camp Lejeune Water Contamination Linked to Birth Defects." *Reuters,* December 6.

U.S. Environmental Protection Agency, Criminal Investigation Division. 2005. "Summary of Investigation, Marine Corps Base Camp Lejeune."

n.d. *Vapor Intrusion Mitigation System(VIMS) Performance Monitoring...* Charlotte, N.C.: CH2M HILL, Inc.

Water, Camp Lejeune: Historic Drinking. n.d. *Timeline.* email: clwater@usmc.mil, Marine Corps.

1996. *Wikipedia.* February 16.

Deadly S.N.A.F.U.

Wikipedia. n.d.

wikipedia. n.d.
"https://en.wikipedia.org/wiki/List_of_2nd_Marine_Divisio

_commanders."